DIABETIC
Cooking For One
Balanced Meals Designed Especially for the Solo Diabetic

D0543858

In the same series
COOKING FOR YOUR DIABETIC CHILD
THE DIABETIC'S MICROWAVE COOKBOOK
PACKED LUNCHES AND SNACKS

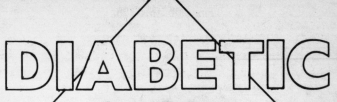

DIABETIC
Cooking For One
Balanced Meals Designed Especially for the Solo Diabetic

Sue Hall

Home Economist to the British Diabetic Association
(1984-86)

THORSONS PUBLISHING GROUP

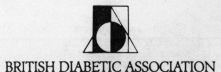

BRITISH DIABETIC ASSOCIATION

First published 1987

© BRITISH DIABETIC ASSOCIATION 1987

Illustrations by Juliet Breese

The British Library Cataloguing in Publication Data

Hall, Sue
Diabetic cooking for one.
1. Diabetes — Diet therapy — Recipes
I. Title
641.5'6314   RC662

ISBN 0-7225-1362-3

Published by Thorsons Publishers Limited,
Wellingborough, Northamptonshire, NN8 2RQ, England

Printed in Great Britain by
Richard Clay Limited, Bungay, Suffolk

3 5 7 9 10 8 6 4

Acknowledgements

The author would like to acknowledge the help of Miss Judith Fishwick with recipe testing, and Andy for testing and constructive criticism.

Contents

		Page
	Introduction	9
1.	Menu Planning for One	15
2.	Microwaving	19
3.	Slow Cooking and Pressure Cooking	36
4.	Economical Use of the Oven	49
5.	No-Cook Recipes	61
6.	Using the Hob and Grill	74
7.	Menu Suggestions	97
	Appendix — Food Values List	101
	Recommended Reading	105
	Further Information	107
	Index	111

Recipes

Throughout the book I have used this standard conversion chart:

Weights	Liquid Measures
25g — 1 oz	150ml — ¼ pint
50g — 2 oz	275ml — ½ pint
75g — 3 oz	425ml — ¾ pint
100g — 4 oz	550ml — 1 pint
150g — 5 oz	
175g — 6 oz	
200g — 7 oz	**Spoon Measures**
225g — 8 oz	1 teaspoon — 5ml
250g — 9 oz	1 dessertspoon — 10ml
275g — 10 oz	1 tablespoon — 15ml
300g — 11 oz	
350g — 12 oz	
375g — 13 oz	
400g — 14 oz	
425g — 15 oz	
450g — 16 oz	

It is best to use this to get accurate results.

Comparative Oven Temperatures are given below:

Oven Temperatures

Fahrenheit	Centigrade	Gas
300°	150°	No 2
325°	160°	No 3
350°	180°	No 4
375°	190°	No 5
400°	200°	No 6
425°	220°	No 7
450°	230°	No 8

Introduction

Most people have to cook a meal just for themselves now and again and many live and cook alone all the time. Cooking for yourself when you have diabetes need not be difficult and is very important. It is vital to ensure that you eat well and choose your foods wisely. The problem with cooking for one is that it is an effort not to have the same thing day in day out, or to rely too heavily on quick or instant foods which may not be so healthy. Cooking and eating for yourself should be a rewarding and pleasant experience; just making a little bit of effort can mean interesting meals and a balanced and healthy diet.

Diabetes needs care and attention, whether you are on insulin, tablets or diet alone. All diabetics on medication should consider carbohydrates and/or calories and even those on diet alone benefit from considering and following general food targets. If you have a dietary allowance you really must try and keep to it. If you are having problems or haven't seen a dietition for a while, or if you are stuck with an allowance which was set many years ago and now doesn't suit your life style or your needs, go back to your clinic or family doctor and ask to see a dietitian. The dietitian can tailor the diet to your needs and give you the help and support you deserve.

Understanding your own diabetes is vital if you are going to achieve good control, which is important in keeping you healthy and feeling fit. Your diet is as important as medication (tablets or insulin) in keeping your blood sugar (glucose) levels down. The purpose of this book is to encourage you to choose wisely and to eat well. Remember that your recommended diet of more fibre/less fat and sugar is a healthy way for everyone to eat. In the reading list on page 105 you will see some useful references to books which explain more about diabetes and its control.

More About Your Food Plan

Why do we place so much emphasis on fibre and fat? A high fibre intake is good for everyone's general health but it is also particularly helpful for diabetics in keeping their blood sugar (glucose) levels more stable. Carbohydrate foods, which are high in fibre, are digested more slowly and the sugar into which they are broken down is released more slowly into the bloodstream than when highly processed foods, or those containing less fibre, are eaten. This slower release into the bloodstream helps to prevent the peaks (highs) and troughs (lows or hypos) in blood sugars, which are dangerous for the diabetic. Another bonus is that the level of fat in the blood is generally lower if you have a high fibre diet. This is good because it is likely to decrease the risk of heart attacks/strokes or problems with circulation.

Selecting a diet with less fat (especially animal fat) is healthier for everyone, because of the connection between high fat intake and heart disease. Diabetics have an increased risk of such problems, so it seems only sensible to strive for a lower animal fat and total fat intake.

These recipes are therefore designed to be as high in fibre and low in fat as possible and can be fitted into most general food plans. Your eating plan or diet will have already emphasized the quantities of food you need to eat, but the types of foods are just as important. As you will see from the traffic lights illustration, we split food choices into green, amber and red, or poor, better and best choices. The recipes here are all designed to encourage you to choose the correct types of foods but there are several basic guidelines to help in everyday cooking.

1. Always trim fat from meat and think about reducing the portion of meat suggested in most cookery books. On average, a 4-5 oz (100-150g) portion of raw meat is adequate for most people. See if you can manage to cook your meat in time to let it go cold, so you can skim off any fat that comes to the surface.

2. Try, where possible, not to add fat during cooking. If you really

have to brown meat, try doing so in a very little vegetable oil in a heavy based or non-stick pan. Always use a minimum of fat. Remember to grill instead of frying. Use a rack in your oven when cooking meat and always use a rack in the microwave.

3.   Try only to use skimmed milk when you cook and look for skimmed milk cheeses instead of cream cheese whenever possible. Skimmed and semi-skimmed milk have the same carbohydrate value as whole milk, but obviously less fat and less calories. UHT or Long Life milk have the same carbohydrate and calorie content as its fresh counterpart.

4.   Use very little butter or margarine. Try to use a reduced fat spread. If possible always choose fats of a vegetable origin.

5.   Try to use wholemeal flour to thicken your sauces and in your baking and pastry.

6.   Try to use brown rice and wholemeal pasta in place of the normal white variety.

7.   Add cooked or tinned beans to casseroles, pies etc. Every ounce of beans you use adds only 5 grammes of carbohydrate and approximately 25 calories, but it is an important source of fibre in your meal. If an ordinary recipe specifies tinned beans but you don't have any, 5-6 oz (150-175g) of dried beans soaked and cooked will replace a large 15oz (425g) tin of beans, and therefore you should be able to work out from that how much you need for the recipe. There is no need to worry about beans which mention sugar on their label, as only a tiny quantity is used and most of it is lost when you rinse and drain your beans. If you are going to use dried beans then you must remember to soak them overnight or bring them to the boil and soak them for two hours. The beans must then be cooked as instructed. It is important that all dried beans are boiled for at least ten minutes before going on to be cooked. Remember: tinned or cooked beans freeze well and keep well in the fridge, as long as they are covered.

8.   If you are buying tinned fish, make sure you buy a variety which is tinned in brine or tomato sauce rather than oil, and if you are

buying tinned fruit, look for fruit which is tinned in natural juice.

Choosing Your Foods

It's best to think of your foods in three groups:

   (a) best choices;
   (b) satisfactory choices;
   (c) poor choices.

(a)   The best choice foods should make up most of your meals and are foods like: wholemeal or wholewheat bread, wholewheat pasta, brown rice, all vegetables and fruits (fresh, frozen without sugar or tinned in natural juice or low calorie syrup), lean meat, fish, reduced-fat spreads, low fat cheese, and skimmed milk.

(b)   The satisfactory choice foods should be used with care and not as often as the above foods. They are things like: white bread and other white flour products, prepared pies, pasties and savoury flans, fatty meat, pâtés and spreads, full fat dairy products such as hard or spreading cheeses, margarine, butter, nuts, and alcoholic drinks.

(c)   The poor choices should be avoided as much as possible — they are for very special occasions or emergencies. They are foods like: sugar, glucose, very sugary foods, sweets, chocolate, fruits tinned in syrup, sweetened drinks, rich cakes and pastries, prepared sweetened puddings, and instant desserts.

You can think of your choices as traffic lights if you find it easier:
GREEN *for foods you should use:*
AMBER *for foods you can use with caution;*
RED *for foods which shouldn't be used regularly but may be used on special occasions.*

RED — STOP

Don't use these foods except on
special occasions.

AMBER — CAUTION

Use these foods with care and
not as the largest part of the diet.

GREEN — GO

Use these foods regularly.

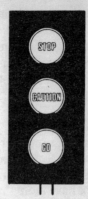

The Recipes

Freezing notes are added to recipes to help your planning. All spoon
measures are level and you should use *either* the Imperial *or* the Metric
measurements, not mix the two. When clingfilm is used in the
microwave section, it is recommended that it does not come into
contact with the food. All the recipes of course are thoroughly tried
and tested. Some of the recipes use ingredients you may not have
met before, so the following notes might be helpful.

Flour
(a) Wholemeal and Wholemeal Self-Raising. These are 100%
wholemeal flour made from the whole grain. They contain lots of
fibre and are very useful for baking and for use in sauces. They also
make good pastry. The self-raising version should always be used
if it is specified in the recipe.

(b) 81% Plain and Self-Raising. The figure 81% refers to the
extraction rate of the flour during milling, i.e. the amount of grain
left in the flour. These therefore contain less fibre than wholemeal
but more than white flour. They are a good compromise choice and
often produce lighter results than the wholemeal versions. If a recipe
specifies 81% then this should be used. You will affect the result and
of course the figures by changing around flours in recipes. These
flours are made by several companies and are available in health food
shops and many supermarkets.

Low-Fat Spread (Margarine)

Always try to use a low fat spread of vegetable origin e.g. sunflower low-fat spread. These are now widely available in many supermarkets. Some of the recipes mention margarine instead of low-fat spread. If this is specified it should always be used, because the recipe requires it.

Fructose (Fruit Sugar)

This is a bulk sweetener sold under the name of Dietade or Fructofin, in chemists and supermarkets. In our recipes we have followed normal BDA policy of not counting the carbohydrate so long as one does not have more than 1 oz (25g) per day. If you use lots of the recipes in one day you will need to bear in mind the amount of fructose you are eating. The calories in fructose are always counted.

1. Menu Planning for One

'Menu' may seem a rather elegant word to use when talking about planning a meal to cook just for yourself. You do need to understand, however, that all of your food choices are important and if you are going to aim for a total daily intake which is high in fibre and low in fat, you need to plan around the main courses or dishes that you decide to make. I have given a list below of some of the convenience foods which come in small portions and would be considered suitable for use in the diet of a diabetic sometimes. Also, by using the food values list on page 101 and the food values given below, you will be able to put in natural foods to complement these convenience foods. Remember though, just having one low-fat meal or one low-fat dish in the day and then eating lots of high-fat products doesn't balance itself out. We need to think about all the snack and meal choices that we make. On page 97, I have given some suggestions for menus using recipes from the book, but, of course, you can swap and change them to fit in with your own allowances.

Food	Weight/Size	Approx CHO	Cals
Boil-in-bag fish:			
Cod in butter sauce	1 packet	4g	140
Cod in cheese sauce	,,	5g	170
Cod in mushroom			
sauce	,,	4-7g	160-180
Cod in parsley sauce	,,	4-7g	140-160
Cod steak in seafood	6 oz (170g)		
sauce	packet	6g	120

Food	Weight/Size	Approx CHO	Cals
Beefburgers:			
thick	4 oz (100g)	neg	230
thin	2 oz (50g)	neg	80
Chicken fingers	1	7g	60
Low-fat beefburgers,			
when grilled	1	1g	75
Low-fat sausages,			
when grilled	1	3g	55
Shepherds pie	8 oz (227g) tray	21g	270
Corned beef	1 oz (25g)	neg	60
Tuna fish in brine	1 oz (25g)	—	35
Tinned beans, drained	1 oz (25g)	5g	25
Fruit			
Apples, eating, whole	1	10g	40
Apricots, fresh, whole	3 medium	10g	40
Bananas, with skin	Small	10g	40
Blackberries, raw	5 oz (150g)	10g	45
Cherries, fresh, whole	4 oz (100g)	10g	40
Dates:			
fresh, whole	3	10g	40
dried, without stones	3	10g	40
Grapes, whole	3 oz (75g)	10g	40
Melon, all types,			
weighed with skin	Large slice	10g	40
Nectarine, fresh, whole	1	10g	40
Orange, fresh, whole	1 large	10g	40
Peach, fresh, whole	1	10g	40
Pears, fresh, whole	1	10g	40
Plums, dessert, fresh,			
whole	4 oz (100g)	10g	40
Prunes, dried, without			
stones	1 oz (25g)	10g	40
Raspberries, fresh	6 oz (175g)	10g	45
Strawberries, fresh	5 oz (150g)	10g	40

Food	Weight/Size	Approx CHO	Cals
Vegetables			
Beetroot, cooked, whole	4 oz (100g)	10g	45
Lentils, dry, raw	1 oz (25g)	10g	60
Peas, marrowfat			
or processed	3 oz (175g)	10g	60
Potatoes:			
raw or boiled	2 oz (50g)	10g	45
chips, cooked	1 oz (25g)	10g	55
jacket, with skin	2 oz (50g)	10g	45
mashed	2 oz (50g)	10g	80
roast	1½ oz (40g)	10g	65

The vegetables listed above are only those which have high enough carbohydrate or calories to make them worth 'counting'. Many vegetables contain very little carbohydrate or calories. An average helping of any of those listed below will not add more than approximately 5g carbohydrate and 20-25 calories to your diet and therefore do not have to be counted into your diet:

Artichokes, asparagus, aubergine, beans (runner), beansprouts, broccoli. Brussels sprouts, cabbage, carrots, cauliflower, celery, courgettes, cucumber, leeks, lettuce, marrow, mushrooms, mustard and cress, okra (raw), peas (fresh or frozen), peppers, pumpkin, radishes, spinach, spring onions, swede, tomatoes (raw and canned), turnip, watercress.

Hints for Solo Cooking

1. Cook twice as many beans as the recipe suggests and freeze half of them for next time.

2. Look carefully at the recipe you are going to make. If it's a recipe that freezes or stores well, why not make double the quantity and keep some for next time? This will save you having to cook another time.

3. Try and get into the habit of setting the table and taking the time to eat properly. Just grabbing a snack because you are by yourself

makes it difficult to eat well and choose healthy foods.

4.   Take advantage of shops and supermarkets which allow you to buy loose food, such as those where you can choose your own vegetables or buy one burger at a time. This is more helpful for you than buying a great big packet, because it means the food will be fresher. Don't be frightened to ask the butcher for just one chop or a couple of sausages. There is no reason to feel pressurized if you aren't spending a lot of money.

5.   It may sometimes be easier for you to use bought or convenience products because you don't want to cook just for yourself. I have therefore given details of suitable convenience foods in the section on meal planning but it is important to realize that you need to plan carefully when you use these foods and not use them exclusively.

6.   Plan ahead. Look at the recipe you have chosen — if it uses half an onion or green pepper, find another recipe to use the other half. Shop for both recipes and cook the second one later in the week. On some of the recipes I have made notes to help you match up dishes and save time.

7.   If a recipe calls for a medium tomato and you don't have a fresh one, use 1 heaped tablespoon of chopped tinned tomatoes. Store the rest sealed (not in their tin) in the fridge or freezer.

8.   Plan your meals so that everything is cooked in the oven or on the hob to save you putting the oven on for one dish.

2. Microwaving

Pork and Butter Bean Casserole

Serves 1	Total CHO — 20g	Total Cals — 215

3 oz (75g) lean
pork, cubed
1 clove of garlic,
crushed
2 oz (50g) canned
butter beans,
drained
1 small carrot, sliced
1 small parsnip,
sliced
¼ pint (150ml)
chicken stock
1 × 5 oz (150g) can
tomatoes

1. Place all the ingredients in a bowl, cover with cling film and pierce the top.
2. Microwave on HIGH for 3 minutes. Stir, replace cling film and cook on HIGH for 15 minutes.
3. Allow to stand for 10 minutes.

Note: This recipe freezes well.

Mushroomed Pork

Serves 1	Total CHO — 10g	Total Cals — 185

3 oz (75g) lean
pork, cubed
3 oz (75g) button
mushrooms, sliced
2 tablespoons canned
sweetcorn
2 teaspoons
wholemeal flour
2 tablespoons
natural yogurt
A little garlic salt
¼ pint (150ml) stock

1. Place all the ingredients in a bowl. Stir well, cover with cling film and pierce the top.

2. Microwave on HIGH for 3 minutes. Stir and replace cling film.

3. Microwave on HIGH for 15 minutes. Allow to stand for 10 minutes.

Note: This recipe freezes well.

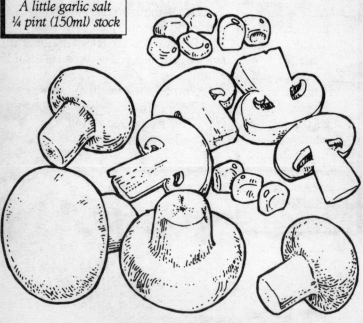

Casseroled Pork

Serves 1	Total CHO — 10g	Total Cals — 180

*4 oz (100g) leeks,
washed and sliced
1 teaspoon vegetable
oil
3 oz (75g) shoulder
of pork, cubed
2 teaspoons
wholemeal flour
¼ pint (150ml)
brown ale
1 oz (25g) mushrooms
1 teaspoon mixed
herbs
Sea salt and freshly
ground black pepper*

1. Microwave the leeks in oil on HIGH for 2 minutes.
2. Toss meat in flour, add to leeks, cover with cling film and pierce the top.
3. Microwave on HIGH for 3 minutes.
4. Add remaining ingredients. Replace cling film and microwave on HIGH for 15 minutes. Allow to stand for 10 minutes.

Note: This recipes freezes well.

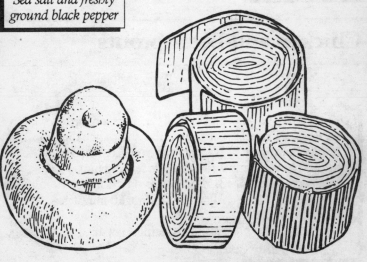

Chicken and Vegetables

Serves 1   Total CHO — 5g   Total Cals — 150

1 chicken breast
(about 4 oz/100g)
1 small onion,
chopped
1 small carrot,
chopped
½ small green pepper,
chopped
¼ pint (150ml)
chicken stock
2 tablespoons dry
white wine (optional)
Seasoning

1. Place all the ingredients in a bowl, cover with cling film and pierce the top.
2. Microwave on HIGH for 3 minutes. Stir well and replace cling film.
3. Microwave on HIGH for 10 minutes. Allow to stand for 10 minutes.

Note: This recipe freezes well.

Chicken and Beansprouts

Serves 1   Total CHO — 10g   Total Cals — 165

1 chicken breast (about
4 oz/100g), skinned
2 oz (50g) sweetcorn
3 oz (75g) beansprouts
½ teaspoon ground
ginger
¼ pint (150ml)
chicken stock
Seasoning

1. Place all the ingredients in a bowl, cover with cling film and pierce the top.
2. Microwave on HIGH for 3 minutes. Stir well and replace cling film.
3. Microwave on HIGH for 10 minutes. Allow to stand for 10 minutes.

Note: This recipe is *not* suitable for freezing.

Fish 'n' Beans

Serves 1	Total CHO — 15g	Total Cals — 120

*1 lean cod fillet
(about 6oz/175g)
2 oz (50g) fresh/frozen
green beans
1 oz (25g) sweetcorn
½×10 oz (275g) can
mushroom soup*
½ medium onion,
chopped
Sea salt and freshly
ground black pepper
3 fl oz (75ml) water*

1. Place all the ingredients in a large bowl. Cover with cling film and pierce the top.
2. Microwave on HIGH for 10 minutes. Allow to stand for 10 minutes.

Note: This recipe freezes well.

* Use the other half for lunch one day with a wholemeal roll and salad!

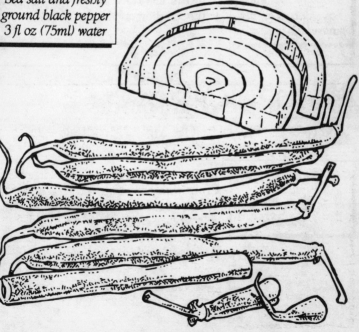

Mexican Liver

Serves 1   Total CHO — 15g   Total Cals — 255

---

2 oz (50g) lamb's liver,
    finely sliced
1 dessertspoon
    vegetable oil
½ medium onion
½×5 oz (150g) can
    red kidney beans *
2 medium tomatoes,
    sliced
3 tablespoons water
Sea salt and freshly
ground black pepper

1. Place the liver, oil and onion in a bowl.
2. Cover with cling film and pierce the top.
Microwave on HIGH for 3 minutes.
3. Stir in remaining ingredients, replace
cling film and microwave on HIGH for 10
minutes. Allow to stand for 10 minutes.

Note: This recipe freezes well.

* Add the rest to a salad or freeze them until
you need them again.

Pasta in Your Microwave

Serves 1   Total CHO — 35g   Total Cals — 160

---

2 oz (50g) wholegrain
    pasta
¼ pint (150ml) boiling
    water

1. Pour water over pasta in a large bowl.
Cover with cling film and pierce the top.
2. Microwave on HIGH for 3 minutes. Stir
and replace cling film.
3. Microwave on HIGH for 3 minutes.
Allow to stand for 5 minutes.

Note: This recipe is not suitable for freezing.

Last-Minute Pasta

Serves 1   Total CHO — 40g   Total Cals — 290

1 clove of garlic,
  crushed
2 rashers very lean
bacon, trimmed and
  chopped
½ green pepper,
  chopped
2 oz (50g) button
mushrooms, sliced
A knob of low-fat
  spread
½ small carton low-fat
  natural yogurt
2 oz (50g) wholegrain
pasta, cooked
  (see page 24)

1. Place all the ingredients, except the yogurt and pasta, in a bowl.
2. Microwave on HIGH for 4 minutes. Top pasta with vegetable mixture, pour on yogurt and serve.

Note: This recipe is *not* suitable for freezing.

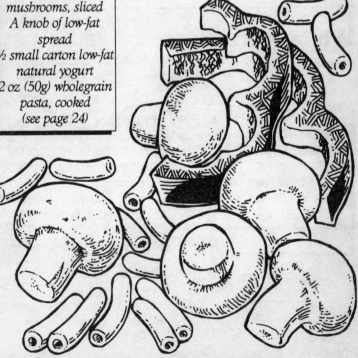

Rice in Your Microwave

Serves 1   Total CHO — 45g   Total Cals — 210

---

2 oz (50g) long grain brown rice
¼ pint (150ml) boiling water

1. Pour water over rice in a large bowl. Stir, cover with cling film and pierce the top.
2. Microwave on HIGH for 4 minutes. Stir well and replace cling film.
3. Microwave on HIGH for 2 minutes. Allow to stand for 5 minutes.

Note: This recipe is *not* suitable for freezing.

White Sauce

Serves 1   Total CHO — 15g   Total Cals — 190

½ oz (15g) polyunsaturated margarine
1 tablespoon wholemeal flour
¼ pint (150ml) skimmed milk

1. Place the margarine and flour together in a jug. Blend together well.
2. Microwave on HIGH for 1 minute.
3. Gradually stir in the milk, a little at a time, mixing thoroughly.
4. Microwave on HIGH for 4 minutes, stirring every minute. Season to taste.

Note: This recipe is *not* suitable for freezing.

Cheese Sauce

Serves 1	Total CHO — 15g	Total Cals — 250

½ oz (15g) polyunsaturated margarine
1 tablespoon wholemeal flour
¼ pint (150ml) skimmed milk
1 oz (25g) reduced-fat hard cheese, grated

1. Place margarine and flour together in a jug. Blend together well.
2. Microwave on HIGH for 1 minutes.
3. Gradually stir in milk, mixing thoroughly.
4. Microwave on HIGH for 3 minutes, stirring every minute.
5. Add cheese and stir well. Microwave on HIGH for 1 minute. Season to taste.

Note: This recipe is *not* suitable for freezing.

Jacket Potato

Serves 1	Total CHO — 25g	Total Cals — 110

5 oz (150g) raw potato

1. Scrub the potato and prick well.
2. Cook in the microwave on HIGH for 5 minutes. Leave to stand for 3 minutes.

Note: If the potato is still a little hard, cook for a further minute or until tender.

This recipe is *not* suitable for freezing.

Vegetable Jacket Potato

Serves 1   Total CHO — 30g   Total Cals — 150

---

*1 oz (25g) onion,
chopped
5 oz (150g) raw potato
1 oz (25g) sweetcorn
1 oz (25g) peas*

1. Place onion in a bowl with a very small amount of low-fat spread. Cook on HIGH for 30 seconds.

2. Scrub and prick the potato well.

3. Cook in microwave on HIGH for 5 minutes.

4. Cut the potato in half and scoop out the inside.

5. Mix with the onion, peas and corn.

6. Place back into the potato shell and allow to stand for 3 minutes.

Note: If the potato is still a little hard, cook for a further minute or until tender.

This recipe is *not* suitable for freezing.

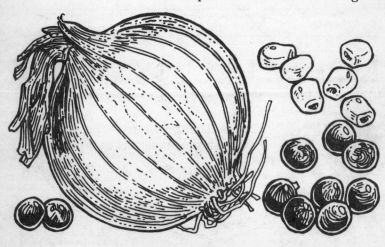

Cheesy Jacket Potato

Serves 1	Total CHO — 25g	Total Cals — 170

5 oz (150g) raw potato
1 oz (25g) reduced-fat
hard cheese, grated

1. Scrub the potato and prick well.
2. Cook in the microwave on HIGH for 5 minutes.
3. Cut the potato in half and scoop out the inside.
4. Mix with the cheese.
5. Place back into the potato shell and allow to stand for 3 minutes.

Note: If the potato is still a little hard, cook for a further minute or until tender.

This recipe is *not* suitable for freezing.

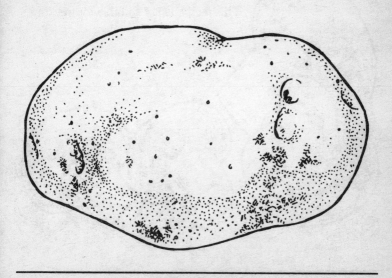

Ham and Mushroom Jacket Potato

Serves 1   Total CHO — 25g   Total Cals — 155

1 oz (25g) mushrooms
5 oz (150g) raw potato
1 oz (25g) cooked
lean ham

1. Peel or wash the mushrooms. Place in a bowl with ½ teaspoon water. Cook for 1 minute in microwave on HIGH.

2. Scrub and prick the potato well.

3. Cook in the microwave on HIGH for 5 minutes.

4. Cut the potato in half and scoop out the inside.

5. Mix with the mushroom and ham.

6. Place back into the potato shell and allow to stand for 3 minutes.

Note: If the potato is still a little hard, cook for a further minute or until tender.

This recipe is *not* suitable for freezing.

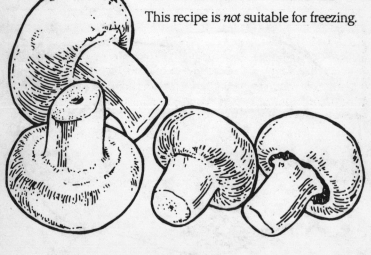

Boiled Potatoes

Serves 1   Total CHO — 20g   Total Cals — 85

---

4 oz (100g) raw potato

1. Peel and wash the potatoes.
2. Cut into even-sized pieces.
3. Place in a bowl with 1 tablespoon water.
4. Cook on HIGH for 3 minutes.

Note: If the potatoes are still hard, cook for a further minute or until tender.

This recipe is *not* suitable for freezing.

Baked Egg Custard

Serves 1   Total CHO — 10g   Total Cals — 130

---

6 fl oz (175ml)
skimmed milk
1×size 3 egg
2 drops of sweetener
Ground nutmeg

1. Beat egg lightly.
2. Stir together milk and sweetener. Microwave on HIGH for 1 minute.
3. Stir the warmed milk into the egg.
4. Pour into a glass.
5. Sprinkle ground nutmeg over the top.
6. Heat on HIGH for 2 minutes.
7. Leave to stand.

Note: This recipe is *not* suitable for freezing.

Fruit Compote

Serves 1   Total CHO — 20g   Total Cals — 80

¼ pint (150ml)
boiling water
liquid sweetener
2 oz (50g) mixed
dried fruit
1 teaspoon cinnamon

1. Place the boiling water in the bowl.
2. Stir in the sweetener, fruit and cinnamon.
3. Cover with cling film. Pierce the top. Heat on HIGH for 3 minutes, take out and stir. Cover with cling film. Pierce the top and heat on HIGH for 4 minutes.
4. Allow to stand for 20-30 minutes for the fruit to rehydrate.
5. Chill before serving.

Note: This recipe is *not* suitable for freezing.

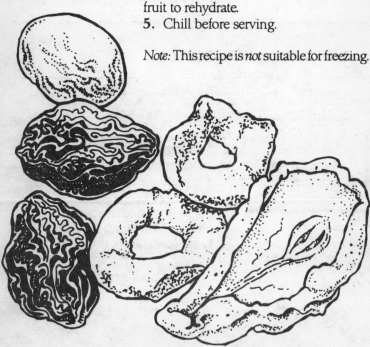

Upside-Down Pudding

Serves 1   Total CHO — 30g   Total Cals — 335

---

1 oz (25g) low-fat spread
½ oz (15g) fructose (fruit sugar)
1 × size 3 egg
1 oz (25g) wholemeal flour
1 oz (25g) dried apricots

1. Cream together the fat and the fructose.
2. Gradually stir in the egg.
3. Fold in the flour.
4. Lay the fruit in the bottom of a small dish.
5. Spread the mixture on top of the fruit.
6. Cook for 4 minutes on HIGH.

Note: This recipe freezes well.

Banana Crunch

Serves 1   Total CHO — 30g   Total Cals — 140

---

1 small banana (2 oz/50g)
1 teaspoon rum
2 tablespoons unsweetened orange juice
1 oz (25g) unsweetened muesli

1. Slice the banana and lay it in the bottom of a small dish.
2. Pour the rum and orange juice on to the banana. Cook on HIGH for 1 minute. Turn the banana and cook on HIGH for a further minute.
3. Sprinkle the muesli on the top and cook for a further minute on HIGH.

Note: This recipe is *not* suitable for freezing.

Baked Stuffed Apple

Serves 1   Total CHO — 20g   Total Cals — 115

---

1 medium cooking
apple
½ oz (15g) currants
1 tablespoon water

1. Remove core from apple. Fill with fruit.
2. Place stuffed apple and water in a dish. Cover with cling film and pierce the top. Microwave on HIGH for 3-4 minutes.

Note: This recipe is *not* suitable for freezing.

Hot Fruit Kebabs

Serves 1   Total CHO — 10g   Total Cals — 40

½ banana, peeled and
sliced
½ red apple, sliced
1 pineapple ring
(canned in natural
juice), drained and
chopped
Lemon juice
Cinnamon

1. Place alternate pieces of prepared fruit on wooden skewers, dividing the fruit evenly between 3 skewers.
2. Mix lemon juice and cinnamon. Brush onto fruit.
3. Place kebabs on a ceramic dish and microwave on HIGH for 2 minutes. Brush again with juice.
4. Microwave for a further 2 minutes. Serve immediately.

Note: This recipe is *not* suitable for freezing.

Ginger Grapefruit

Serves 1   Total CHO — 5g   Total Cals — 25

½ *large grapefruit*
1 teaspoon dried
ginger
Liquid sweetener
to taste

1. Loosen segments of grapefruit. Sprinkle on ginger evenly.
2. Microwave on HIGH for 2 minutes. Sweeten to taste and serve.

Note: This recipe is *not* suitable for freezing.

Fruity Porridge

Serves 1   Total CHO — 25g   Total Cals — 130

---

1 oz (25g) rolled oats
¼ *pint (150ml) boiling*
water
½ *oz (15g) dried*
apricots, soaked and
chopped
1 tablespoon low-fat
natural yogurt

1. Soak the oats in water for 15 minutes. Mix in apricots.
2. Microwave on HIGH for 2 minutes. Stir well. Microwave on HIGH for a further 2 minutes.
3. Allow to stand for 5 minutes. Stir in yogurt and serve.

Note: This recipe is *not* suitable for freezing.

3. Slow Cooking and Pressure Cooking

Slow Bacon and Sweetcorn Soup

Serves 5	Total CHO — 70g	Total Cals — 350

8 oz (225g) potato, peeled and chopped
1 onion, chopped
Sea salt and freshly ground black pepper
Bay leaf
Ground nutmeg
3 tablespoons skimmed milk
1 oz (25g) lean bacon, grilled
1×5 oz (150g) can sweetcorn, drained

1. Place potatoes, onion and seasoning in cooker with just enough water to cover. Cook on HIGH for 3 hours.
2. Add milk, bacon and sweetcorn, stir well and cook for 30 minutes.

Each portion contains 15g CHO and 65 calories.

Note: This recipe freezes well. Serve as a main course or lunch, and freeze the spare portions.

Slow Curried Chicken

Serves 2   Total CHO — 35g   Total Cals — 460

2 chicken portions,
skinned
1 tablespoon
wholemeal flour
Sea salt and freshly
ground black pepper
A dash of oil
1 small onion,
chopped
1 small cooking
apple, peeled and
chopped
1 oz (25g) raisins
2 teaspoons curry
powder
¼ pint (150ml) boiling
water
2 tablespoons natural
yogurt

1. Coat chicken in flour, salt and pepper. Lightly fry in oil. Add vegetables and fry for 5 minutes.

2. Place in slow cooker with all the ingredients except the yogurt. Cook on HIGH for 3-4 hours.

3. Pour on yogurt before serving.

1 portion (1 chicken joint plus half the sauce) contains about 20g CHO and 230 calories.

Note: This recipes freezes well. Make 2 portions and freeze one.

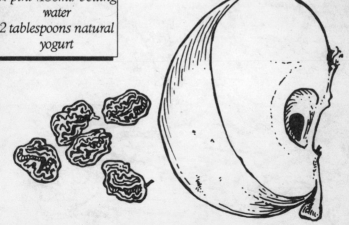

Slow-Cook Oriental Chicken

Serves 1   Total CHO — 10g   Total Cals — 170

A dash of oil
1 chicken breast
(4 oz/100g), skinned
1 medium onion,
chopped
1 teaspoon
wholemeal flour
3 fl oz (75ml) stock
3 oz (75g) mushrooms
1 teaspoon soya sauce
2 oz (50g) beansprouts

1. Heat the oil in a frying pan and brown the chicken.
2. Place all the ingredients in slow cooker and stir well.
3. Cook for 4 hours.

Note: This recipe freezes well.

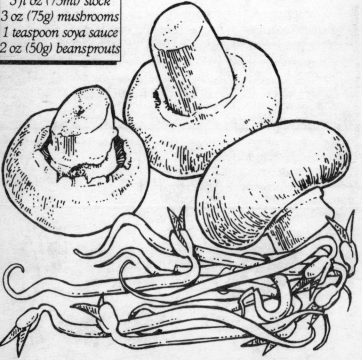

Ratatouille

Serves 1   Total CHO — 10g   Total Cals — 45

A dash of oil
½ medium aubergine,
    sliced
½ medium onion,
    chopped
½ red pepper, sliced
1×5 oz (150g) can
    tomatoes
1 courgette, sliced
Seasoning to taste

1. Fry vegetables gently in oil for 5 minutes.
2. Season and place in cooker. Cook for 5-7 hours.

Note: This recipe freezes well.

Slow-Cook Lime and Ginger Pears

Serves 1   Total CHO — 10g   Total Cals — 50

1 large pear, peeled,
    cored and halved
1 teaspoon ground
    ginger
Rind of 1 lemon
6 fl oz (175ml) low-
calorie/sugar-free lime
    squash
2 tablespoons natural
    yogurt

1. Place pears in base of cooker. Sprinkle with ginger and lemon rind.
2. Pour on squash. Cook for 2-3 hours.
3. Serve with natural yogurt.

Note: This recipe freezes well without the yogurt.

Slow Liver and Onions

Serves 1   Total CHO — 10g   Total Cals — 225

A dash of oil
4 oz (100g) lamb's
liver, sliced
1 tablespoon
wholemeal flour
1 small onion,
chopped
½ pint (275ml) stock

1. Gently heat the oil in a frying pan. Coat the liver in flour and brown it in the oil.
2. Place all the ingredients in the slow cooker and stir well.
3. Cook for 3-4 hours until the meat is tender.

Note: This recipe is *not* suitable for freezing.

Yogurt

Makes 1 pint (550ml)   Total CHO — 35g   Total Cals — 235

1 pint (550ml) semi-
skimmed UHT milk
2 tablespoons natural
yogurt
1 tablespoon dried
skimmed milk

1. Mix all the ingredients well and place in slow cooker.
2. Cover with a tea towel but no lid.
3. Cook for 45 minutes on LOW. Switch off cooker, place lid over tea towel and leave for 2 hours.
4. Stir well, pour into a covered container and chill for 1 hour. Use as required. Stores well in fridge.

Note: This recipe is *not* suitable for freezing.

Quick Chicken Curry and Rice

Serves 1   Total CHO — 60g   Total Cals — 390

A dash of oil
½ small onion,
chopped
1 chicken breast (about
4 oz/100g), skinned
2 teaspoons curry
powder
½ pint (275ml) stock
3 dried apricot halves,
soaked for 2 hours
A few sultanas
2 oz (50g) brown rice
¼ pint (150ml) water

1. Brown onion and chicken in oil, add curry powder and stir well.
2. Add stock and fruit. Place trivet over chicken. Line separator with foil and put in rice and water, cover loosely with foil.
3. Bring to high (15lbs) pressure and cook for 5 minutes. Reduce pressure slowly.
4. Rinse and drain rice. Serve. Thicken sauce if necessary with a teaspoon of wholemeal flour.

Note: This recipe freezes well without the rice.

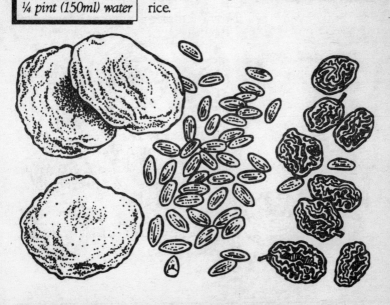

Spicy Pasta Supper

Serves 1	Total CHO — 35g	Total Cals — 290

A dash of oil
3 oz (75g) lean stewing steak, sliced finely
2 teaspoons horseradish sauce
1 teaspoon tomato purée
¼ pint (150ml) stock
2 oz (50g) wholewheat pasta shells
¼ pint (150ml) water

1. Brown the meat in the oil and remove from pan. Mix horseradish sauce, tomato purée and stock.
2. Pour stock into pan. Place trivet over stock with meat on trivet.
3. Bring to high (15lbs) pressure and cook for 10 minutes. Reduce pressure quickly.
4. Line separator with foil, place pasta in separator with water. Place on top of meat.
5. Bring to high (15lbs) pressure and cook for 10 minutes. Reduce pressure slowly.
6. Strain pasta and serve.

Note: The meat part of this dish freezes well.

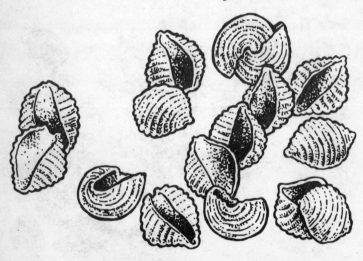

Lemony Chicken

Serves 1	Total CHO — 5g	Total Cals — 150

A dash of oil
1 clove of garlic, crushed
½ small onion, chopped
Mixed dried herbs
1 chicken breast (about 4 oz/100g), skinned
½ pint (275ml) stock
2 tablespoons natural yogurt
2 tablespoons lemon juice

1. Mix the oil, garlic, onion and herbs. Leave to stand.
2. Meanwhile, brown the chicken breast in the open pan, add the oil mixture and the stock.
3. Bring to high (15lbs) pressure and cook for 10 minutes. Reduce pressure quickly. Stir in the yogurt and lemon juice.

Note: This recipe freezes well.

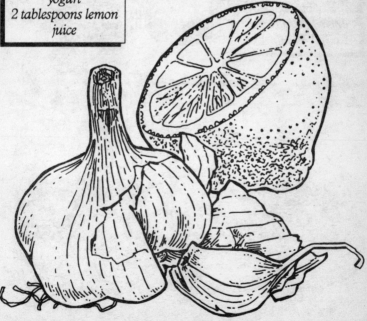

Liver and Borlotti Beans

Serves 1	Total CHO — 15g	Total Cals — 300

2 oz (50g) canned
    borlotti beans
1 large carrot, sliced
½ small onion,
    chopped
1 rasher lean bacon,
    chopped
1 courgette, sliced
4 oz (100g) lamb's
    liver, cubed
A dash of tomato
    purée
Mixed dried herbs
½ pint (275ml) stock

1. Place all ingredients in pan and mix well.

2. Bring to high (15lbs) pressure. Cook for 20 minutes. Reduce pressure quickly.

Note: This recipe freezes well.

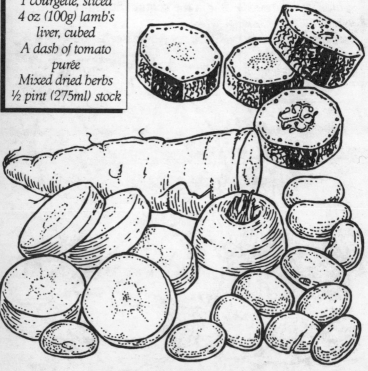

Marmalade Lamb

Serves 1   Total CHO — 10g   Total Cals — 275

A dash of oil
½ small onion,
chopped
1 clove garlic, crushed
1 lean lamb chop, trim
off the fat
½ pint (275ml) stock
1 tablespoon low-
sugar marmalade
1 orange, juice and
grated rind
A handful of almonds

1. Gently fry onion and garlic in oil in open pan.

2. Add chop and brown well.

3. Add remaining ingredients and stir well. Bring to high (15lbs) pressure. Cook for 15 minutes. Reduce pressure quickly.

Note: This recipe freezes well.

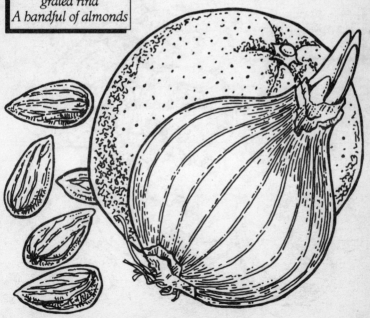

Mushroom Cod

Serves 1	Total CHO — neg	Total Cals — 200

1 rasher very lean
bacon, chopped
A knob of margarine
1 courgette, sliced
1 cod fillet (about
6 oz/175g)
2 oz (50g)
mushrooms, sliced
1×5 oz (150g) can
tomatoes
¼ pint (150ml) water
Seasoning
1 clove of garlic,
crushed

1. In the open pan gently fry the bacon in the margarine for 3 minutes.
2. Add the courgettes and stir well. Add remaining ingredients and stir.
3. Cover pan and bring to high (15lbs) pressure. Cook for 5 minutes. Reduce pressure quickly.

Note: This recipe freezes well.

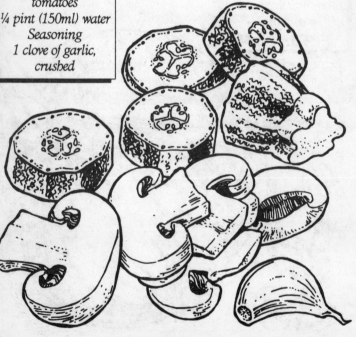

Dried Fruit Salad

Serves 1	Total CHO — 40g	Total Cals — 160

3 oz (75g) mixed dried
fruits
½ pint (275ml)
boiling water
½ teaspoon cinnamon

1. Soak the fruit in the water for 10 minutes.

2. Place all ingredients in pressure cooker. Bring to high (15lbs) pressure and cook for 10 minutes.

3. Reduce pressure slowly.

Note: This recipe is *not* suitable for freezing.

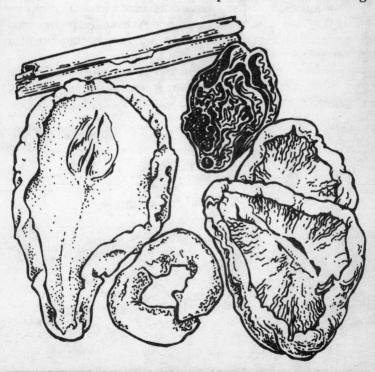

Individual Madeleines

Makes 6   Total CHO — 90g   Total Cals — 1380

4 oz (100g) low-fat
spread
2 oz (50g) fructose
(fruit sugar)
2×size 3 eggs, beaten
4 oz (100g) 81%
self-raising flour
A little warmed
low-sugar jam
2 oz (50g) desiccated
coconut

1. Lightly oil 6 Madeleine tins.

2. Cream fat and fructose until light and fluffy. Beat in eggs, add flour.

3. Divide the mixture evenly between the 6 tins.

4. Place trivet in pressure cooker with 1 pint (550ml) water. Stand tins on trivet and cover with greaseproof paper.

5. Close the cooker and steam gently for 5 minutes. Bring to low (5lbs) pressure and cook for 15 minutes. Reduce pressure slowly.

6. Allow to cool on a wire rack. Remove from tins. Melt jam, brush on to cakes and roll in coconut.

Each cake is 15g CHO and 230 calories.

Note: This recipe freezes well.

4. Economical Use of the Oven

Hot Pot

Serves 1	Total CHO — 25g	Total Cals — 400

4 oz (100g) lean lamb, cubed
1 lamb's kidney, skinned and sliced
1 small carrot, sliced
1 small onion, chopped
3 oz (75g) potato, peeled and sliced
3 fl oz (75ml) stock
2 teaspoons wholemeal flour

1. Put layers of meat and vegetable in a casserole and season to taste. Finish with a layer of thickly sliced potato.
2. Mix stock and flour and pour over meat.
3. Cover and bake at 350°F/180°C (Gas 4) for 1½-2 hours. Uncover casserole for 30 minutes at end of cooking time.

Note: This recipe freezes well.

Sausage Goulash

Serves 1	Total CHO — 20g	Total Cals — 435

2 good quality thick
  pork sausages
½ medium apple,
  sliced
½ medium onion,
  chopped
½ green pepper,
  chopped
½ beef stock cube
1×5 oz (150g) can
  tomatoes
2 tablespoons frozen
  peas

1. Place sausages in a small dish. Cover with apple, onion and pepper.
2. Crumble in stock cube. Add tomatoes with juice from tin.
3. Cover and bake at 400°F/100°C (Gas 6) for 50 minutes. Add peas and cook for another 10 minutes.

Note: This recipe freezes well.

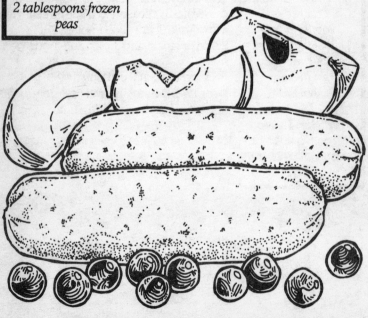

Spicy Pork Chop

Serves 1	Total CHO — neg	Total Cals — 230

*1 small pork chop
(about 4 oz/100g)
Pinch of ground ginger
1 dessertspoon chilli
sauce
1 dessertspoon
Worcester sauce
Pinch of Candarel or
Sweetex
1 dessertspoon vinegar
1 dessertspoon ketchup
1 dessertspoon soya
sauce
1 clove garlic, crushed*

1. Trim the pork chop and rub ginger over it.

2. Cover with foil in an ovenproof dish and bake at 350°F/190° (Gas 5) for 10 minutes.

3. Meanwhile, mix together all remaining ingredients. Pour sauce over chop and re-cover.

4. Bake for 30 minutes.

Note: This recipe freezes well.

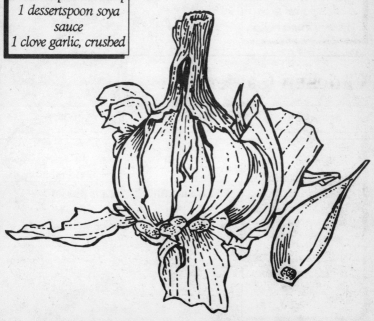

West Country Chop

Serves 1   Total CHO — 5g   Total Cals — 260

1 lean pork chop,
trimmed (about
4 oz/100g)
1 small onion
1 carrot, sliced
Dried mixed herbs
2 oz (50g) turnip,
peeled and diced
¼ pint (150ml) dry
cider
1 tablespoon tomato
purée
3 fl oz (75ml) water

1. Brown the chop gently in a non-stick saucepan, add onion, carrot and turnip. Cook for 2 minutes.
2. Add remaining ingredients and place in a covered dish. Cook at 350°F/180°C (Gas 4) for 1 hour or until chop is tender.

Note: This recipe freezes well.

Chicken Casserole

Serves 1   Total CHO — 5g   Total Cals — 150

1 chicken breast (about
4 oz/100g), boned and
skinned
3 fl oz (75ml) stock
3 fl oz (75ml) dry
white wine
1 oz (25g) mushrooms
½ medium onion,
chopped
½ carrot, chopped

1. Place all the ingredients in a covered casserole. Cook at 400°F/200°C (Gas 6) for ¾-1 hour until chicken is tender.

Note: This recipe freezes well.

Spiced Chicken Fillet

Serves 1	Total CHO — 10g	Total Cals — 185

1 chicken fillet (about
  4 oz/100g), skinned
  and boned
½ medium onion,
  finely chopped
2 oz (50g) green peas
1 small carrot, sliced
3 fl oz (75ml) tomato
  juice
1 tablespoon dry white
  wine
½ teaspoon curry
  powder
½ teaspoon marjoram
Sea salt and freshly
ground black pepper

1. Divide the chicken into two portions and place at the bottom of a casserole dish.
2. Place all the other ingredients on top, cover and bake at 350°F/180°C (Gas 4) for 1 hour. Serve with a garnish of chopped parsley.

Note: This recipe freezes well.

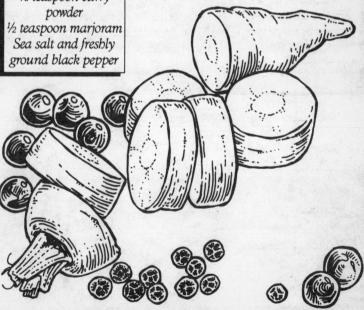

Yogurt Chicken

Serves 1   Total CHO — 10g   Total Cals — 155

3 oz (75g) chicken,
skinned, boned and
sliced
½ medium onion,
finely sliced
3 fl oz (75ml) tomato
juice
½ clove garlic, crushed
½ teaspoon curry
powder
½ teaspoon ground
cardamom
Sea salt and freshly
ground black pepper
½ × 5 oz (150ml)
carton low-fat natural
yogurt *

1. Place the chicken in a casserole dish.
2. Mix together the remaining ingredients, except the yogurt, and pour over the top.
3. Cover and leave to marinade for 24 hours.
4. Bake at 325°F/170°C (Gas 4) for 1 hour. Remove from the oven and stir in the yogurt. Serve hot with green vegetables.

Note: This recipe freezes well.

*Use the other half for your cereal or mixed with chopped fruit for a light dessert, or in Kipper Kedgeree (opposite).

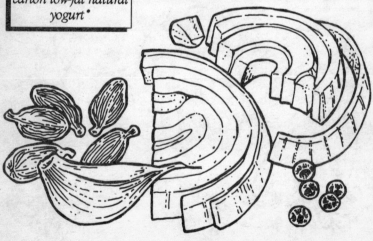

Kipper Kedgeree

Serves 1	Total CHO — 20g	Total Cals — 155

*1 oz (25g) low-fat
spread
4 oz (100g) cooked
kipper fillet, flaked
1×size 3 egg, hard
boiled and chopped
1 oz (25g) brown rice,
cooked (see page 00)
2 tablespoons low-fat
natural yogurt
Seasoning to taste*

1. Melt the low-fat spread, add flaked kipper and eggs.
2. Stir in rice and yogurt, season to taste. Place in an ovenproof dish, cover and bake at 375°F/190°C (Gas 5) for 15-20 minutes. Serve.

Note: This recipe is *not* suitable for freezing.

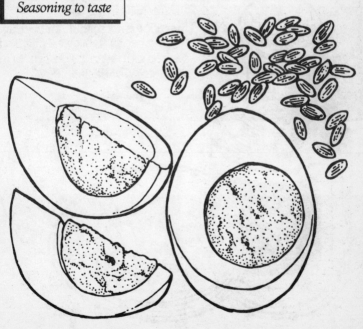

Caramel Custard

Serves 1   Total CHO — 5g   Total Cals — 125

*1 teaspoon fructose
(fruit sugar)
1 tablespoon water
4 fl oz (100ml)
skimmed milk
A drop of vanilla
essence
1 × size 3 egg*

1. Place fructose and water in a small pan. Heat until syrupy and brown. Pour into a ramekin dish.

2. Mix milk and essence and heat to boiling point. Pour onto lightly beaten egg and mix well. Pour into dish.

3. Put a little water in a baking tin and place ramekin in this. Bake at 300°F/150°C (Gas 2) for 30 minutes. Chill and turn out to serve.

Note: This recipe is *not* suitable for freezing.

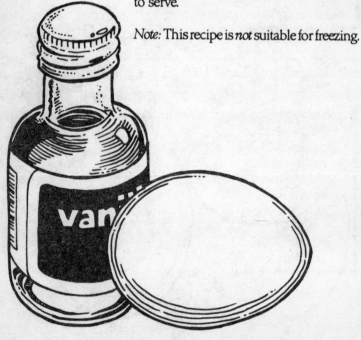

Juicy Bananas

Serves 1   Total CHO — 20g   Total Cals — 75

½ oz (15g) raisins
1 dessertspoon lemon
juice
1 dessertspoon orange
juice
1 medium banana,
peeled

1. Soak raisins in juices for 30 minutes.
2. Place the split banana in a casserole, sprinkle over the raisins and juice. Cover.
3. Bake at 300°F/150°C (Gas 2) for 15 minutes.

Note: This recipe freezes well.

Brown Betty

Serves 1   Total CHO — 30g   Total Cals — 230

1 small eating apple,
peeled and chopped
Juice and rind of 1
small orange
1 oz (25g) self-raising
wholemeal flour
1 oz (25g) low-fat
spread
1 teaspoon Candarel
or Sweetex

1. Place fruit in base of ramekin.
2. Mix topping ingredients well and sprinkle over fruit.
3. Bake at 350°F/180°C (Gas 4) for 20 minutes.

Note: This recipe freezes well.

Apple and Blackberry Crumble

Serves 1   Total CHO — 30g   Total Cals — 240

*1 small eating apple,
peeled and chopped
2 oz (50g) frozen/fresh
blackberries
1 oz (25g) self-raising
wholemeal flour
1 oz (25g) low-fat
spread
1 teaspoon fructose
(fruit sugar)*

1. Place fruit in base of ramekin dish.
2. Mix topping ingredients and sprinkle over fruit.
3. Bake at 350°F/180°C (Gas 4) for 20 minutes.

Note: This recipe freezes well.

Apple Charlotte

Serves 1   Total CHO — 20g   Total Cals — 100

*5 oz (150g) cooking
apples
1 oz (25g) wholemeal
breadcrumbs
Diamin or Candarel
sweetener to taste*

1. Peel, core, chop and stew apples in a little water. When cool, sweeten to taste.
2. Layer wholemeal breadcrumbs and apple in a small ovenproof dish in 4 layers.
3. Bake for 20 minutes at 375°F/190°C (Gas 5) until surface breadcrumbs are brown and crispy.

Serving suggestions: Serve cold with natural yogurt or hot with custard. Remember to add the figure to your dessert.

Note: This recipe freezes well.

Bread and Butter Pudding

Serves 2   Total CHO — 25g   Total Cals — 220

1 large thin slice
wholemeal bread, cut
into 4
A knob of low-fat
spread
½ tablespoon
sultanas
Rind of half of a
lemon, grated
A sprinkling of flaked
almonds
½ pint (275ml)
skimmed milk
1×size 3 egg

1. Thinly spread the bread with low-fat spread.
2. Mix sultanas, lemon rind and half the almonds together.
3. Arrange alternate layers of bread and fruit mixture in a small casserole dish.
4. Beat egg into milk. Pour over bread. Sprinkle on remaining almonds.
5. Bake at 375°F/180°C (Gas 4) for 30 minutes.

Note: This recipe is not suitable for freezing.

Traditional Rice Pudding

Serves 1   Total CHO — 20g   Total Cals — 120

1 tablespoon brown
rice
6 fl oz (175ml)
skimmed milk
Liquid sweetener

1. Put the milk and rice in a small ovenproof bowl.
2. Cover with foil and bake in a moderate oven until tender — about 2 hours. Allow to cool slightly before sweetening.

Note: This recipe is not suitable for freezing.

Bakewell Tart

Makes 2 portions	Total CHO — 40g	Total Cals — 820

2 tablespoons
wholemeal flour
2 tablespoons plain
flour
Pinch of salt
2 tablespoons low-fat
spread
Cold water

For the filling
2 oz (50g) low-fat
spread
2 oz (50g) fructose
(fruit sugar)
1×size 2 egg
1 tablespoon ground
almonds
2 tablespoons
ground rice
Almond essence
1 tablespoon
sugar-free jam

1. Make up the pastry in the usual way and use to line a 4-inch (10cm) flan ring.
2. Place on a baking sheet, cover, fill with baking beans and bake blind for 10 minutes at 400°F/200°C (Gas 6).
3. Melt the low-fat spread and stir in the fructose, add the egg, ground almonds, rice and almond essence, stir well and then allow to cool slightly.
4. Spread the jam on the base of the flan and pour the filling on top. Bake for approximately 15-20 minutes at 400°F/200°C (Gas 6) until well risen and golden brown.
5. Remove the flan ring and cool on a wire tray. Use half and freeze half or store until the next day.

Each portion (½ tart) contains 20g CHO and 205 calories.

Note: This recipe freezes well.

5. No-Cook Recipes

Waldorf Cheese Salad

Serves 1	Total CHO — 10g	Total Cals — 240

4 oz (100g) reduced-fat
    soft cheese
2 oz (50g) apple,
    chopped
1 tablespoon walnuts,
    chopped
2 oz (50g) celery,
    chopped

Mix all the ingredients together well. Chill and use as required.

Note: This recipe is *not* suitable for freezing.

Corn, Pepper and Beansprout Salad

Serves 1	Total CHO — 25g	Total Cals — 145

4 oz (100g)
beansprouts
2 oz (50g)
mushrooms, chopped
8 radishes, sliced
1 small carrot, grated
3 oz (75g) sweetcorn
1 small green pepper,
deseeded and chopped
1 tablespoon low-fat
natural yogurt

Mix all the ingredients together well. Chill and serve.

Note: This recipe is *not* suitable for freezing.

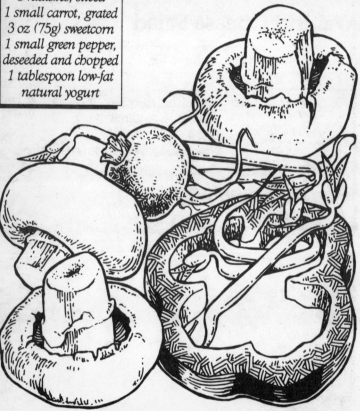

Concertina Tomato

Serves 1	Total CHO — 5g	Total Cals — 220

1 large steak tomato
1 hard-boiled egg (size 2) in 6 slices
2 oz (50g) reduced-fat hard cheese
2 oz (50g) thinly sliced cucumber

Dressing
1 tablespoon lemon juice
1 tablespoon freshly chopped mint

1. Chop 6 horizontal slices into the tomato and put a slice of egg in each slice. Cut cheese into 3 slices and cut into 6 triangles.
2. Put a triangle in each slice of the tomato.
3. Put sections of cucumber behind cheese and egg. Sprinkle with dressing.

Note: This recipe is *not* suitable for freezing.

Chinese Vegetable Salad

Serves 1	Total CHO — 5g	Total Cals —10

2 oz (50g) beansprouts, chopped roughly
1 oz (25g) red pepper, chopped
1 oz (25g) mushrooms, chopped
Dash of soya sauce

Mix all the ingredients together well. Chill and serve.

Note: This recipe needs to be used the day it is made.

It is *not* suitable for freezing.

Tuna and Sweetcorn Salad

Serves 1	Total CHO — 15g	Total Cals — 210

1×4 oz (100g) can of
tuna in brine, drained
1 small onion, finely
chopped
Juice of half a lemon
2 oz (50g) canned
sweetcorn, drained
½ medium red pepper
Sea salt and freshly
ground black pepper
2 tablespoons reduced-
oil mayonnaise

1. Flake the tuna fish and combine with the other salad ingredients.
2. Fold in the mayonnaise and set aside to chill in the refrigerator before serving.

Note: This recipe is *not* suitable for freezing.

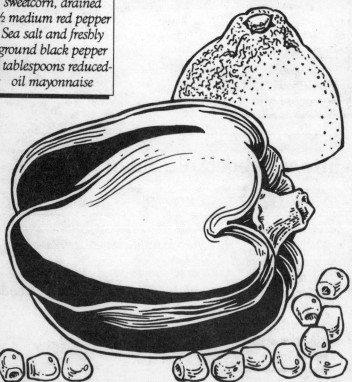

Garlic Chicken Salad

| Serves 1 | Total CHO — 10g | Total Cals — 100 |

2 oz (50g) cooked chicken, diced
1 medium apple, cored and sliced
1 small onion, finely chopped
1 clove of garlic, crushed
Sea salt and freshly ground black pepper
A little oil and vinegar, mixed well

1. Marinade the diced chicken in the oil and vinegar for 2 hours.

2. Add the remaining ingredients. Mix well and serve on a bed of fresh beansprouts.

Note: This recipe is *not* suitable for freezing.

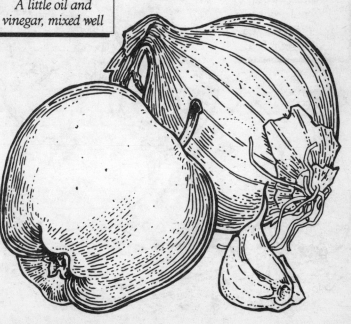

Fruity Beansprout and Chicken Salad

Serves 1	Total CHO — 20g	Total Cals — 315

2 oz (50g) apple, chopped
2 oz (50g) orange
2 oz (50g) beansprouts
½ oz (15g) sultanas
1 oz (25g) almonds, chopped
Lemon juice
4 lettuce leaves, roughly chopped
3 oz (75g) chicken, cooked and diced

1. Mix all the ingredients except chicken together and serve on a bed of lettuce.
2. Place the chicken on top of the salad.

Note: This recipe is *not* suitable for freezing.

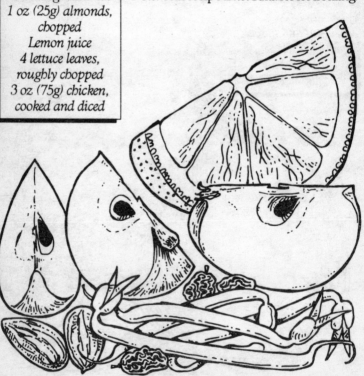

Tuna and Spring Carrot Salad

Serves 1   Total CHO — 10g   Total Cals — 180

2 oz (50g) carrot
1×5 oz (150g) carton
low-fat natural yogurt
2 oz (50g) mushrooms
1 oz (25g) onion
1 tablespoon chopped
fresh parsley
Sea salt and freshly
ground black pepper
3 oz (75g) tuna in
brine, drained

1. Grate the carrot and chop the mushroom and onion finely.
2. Mix together the carrot, yogurt, mushrooms, onion, parsley, salt and pepper.
3. Serve with tuna fish.

Note: This recipe is *not* suitable for freezing.

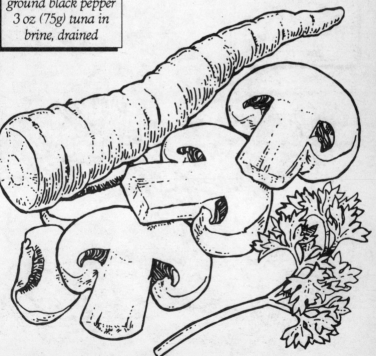

Ham and Haricot Bean Salad

Serves 1	Total CHO — 25g	Total Cals — 330

4 lettuce leaves
5 oz (150g) cooked
haricot beans (or
baked beans with
the tomato sauce
washed off)
Watercress
2 oz (50g) tomato
1 hard-boiled egg
(size 3)
3 oz (75g) cooked
lean ham

1. Slice the egg and place on a bed of lettuce with beans, watercress and chopped tomato and pepper. Season.
2. Serve with ham.

Note: This recipe is *not* suitable for freezing.

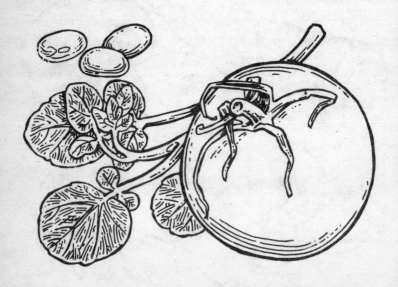

Crunchy Vegetable Mix with Cottage Cheese

Serves 1	Total CHO — 5g	Total Cals — 100

4 lettuce leaves
1 oz (25g) cucumber
2 oz (50g) firm tomato
1 oz (25g) spring onions
1 oz (25g) radish
1 oz (25g) mushrooms
1 oz (25g) green pepper
3 oz (75g) cottage cheese

1. Chop up the cucumber, tomato, spring onions, radish, mushrooms and pepper finely.
2. Lay onto a bed of lettuce leaves.
3. Serve with cottage cheese.

Note: This recipe is *not* suitable for freezing.

Rum, Raisin and Apricot Yogurt

Serves 1	Total CHO — 35g	Total Cals — 170

3 oz (75g) low-fat natural yogurt
½ oz (15g) raisins
½ oz (15g) wheatflakes
1 teaspoon rum
1 oz (25g) dried apricots

1. Chop up the apricots finely.
2. Mix all the ingredients together.

Note: This recipe is *not* suitable for freezing.

Surprise Orange

Serves 1   Total CHO — 10g   Total Cals — 60

---

1 small orange
A few sultanas
½ oz (15g) chopped
nuts

1. Cut the top off the orange (flute the top).
2. Carefully remove the inside fruit.
3. Chop the fruit and mix with the nuts and sultanas.
4. Place the fruit, nuts and sultanas back into the orange shell.
5. Chill and serve.

Note: This recipe is *not* suitable for freezing.

Fruit Crunch

Serves 1   Total CHO — 20g   Total Cals — 175

---

3 oz (75g) low-fat
natural yogurt
½ oz (15g) wholewheat
flakes
½ oz (15g) apricots
½ oz (15g) almonds
or
3 oz (75g) low-fat
natural yogurt
1 oz (25g) muesli
1 oz (25g) apricots

1. Chop up apricots and almonds finely.
2. Mix all the ingredients together.
3. Serve.

The muesli/apricot alternative contains 25g CHO and 155 calories.

Note: This recipe is *not* suitable for freezing.

Fruit Wonder

Serves 1	Total CHO — 5g	Total Cals — 45

2 oz (50g) pear,
chopped
1 oz (25g) cottage
cheese
Liquid sweetener to
taste
Juice of 1 lemon

1. Stir together chopped fruit, cottage cheese, lemon juice and sweetener (to taste).
2. Process in a blender.
3. Pour into a glass and chill.

Note: This recipe is *not* suitable for freezing.

Yogurt Jelly

Serves 2	Total CHO — 10g	Total Cals — 60

½ packet gelatine
3 fl oz (75ml) made-
up sugar-free orange
squash
1×5 oz (150g) carton
diet yogurt

1. Dissolve the gelatine in the squash over a low heat. Allow to cool. Add the yogurt, stirring continuously
2. Mix well. Pour into a small pudding dish and leave to set in the refrigerator. This will take approximately 1½-2 hours.

Note: This recipe is *not* suitable for freezing.

Fruit Fluff

Serves 1	Total CHO — 10g	Total Cals — 60

3 oz (75g) low-fat diet
fruit yogurt
½ egg white
(size 3 egg)

1. Beat the egg white until stiff peaks are formed.
2. Gradually fold the egg white into the yogurt.
3. Chill before serving.

Note: Use the remaining egg white in the ice-cream recipe below.

This recipe is *not* suitable for freezing.

Fruit Yogurt Ice Cream

Serves 1	Total CHO — 10g	Total Cals — 60

3 oz (75g) diet low-fat
fruit yogurt
1 teaspoon fructose
½ egg white
(size 3 egg)

1. Beat the yogurt and fructose.
2. Partly freeze.
3. Fold in the egg white, stiffly beaten.
4. Freeze again.

Note: Use the remaining egg white in the Fruit Fluff recipe above.

This recipe freezes well.

Cheesecake

Serves 1	Total CHO — 20g	Total Cals — 220

*1 oz (25g)
unsweetened muesli
3 oz (75g) curd cheese
Grated rind of half an
orange
1 fl oz (15ml)
unsweetened orange
juice*

1. Sprinkle the muesli onto the base of a small dish.
2. Beat together the cheese, orange rind and juice until smooth.
3. Pour or spoon mixture carefully on muesli base, cover and chill.

Note: This recipe is *not* suitable for freezing.

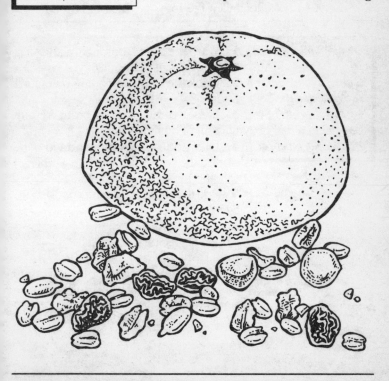

6. Using the Hob and Grill

Beanfeast Soup

Serves 1	Total CHO — 15g	Total Cals — 80

1 oz (25g) mixed dried beans*
½ pint (275ml) water
½ stock cube
1 oz (25g) onion
Sea salt and freshly ground black pepper

1. Wash the beans thoroughly, and soak them for at least 12 hours.
2. Cook the beans in boiling water for 1 hour.
3. Dissolve the stock cube in ½ pint (275ml) of boiling water.
4. Drain the cooked beans and add to the stock cube liquid. Season with a pinch of salt and pepper.
5. Add the onion and simmer until tender. Serve.

Note: This recipe freezes well.

*If mixed beans are unobtainable, buy individual packets of beans and mix to the stated weight.

Pancake Parcels

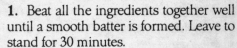

Makes 8	Total CHO — 80g	Total Cals — 485

4 oz (100g)
wholemeal flour
A pinch of sea salt
1×size 3 egg, beaten
½ pint (275ml)
skimmed milk

1. Beat all the ingredients together well until a smooth batter is formed. Leave to stand for 30 minutes.

2. Heat a little oil in a heavy-based pan. Pour a little batter into the pan. After 3-4 minutes, turn and cook other side. When cooked, stack the pancakes separated by layers of greaseproof paper.

3. Fill as desired. Some recipes for fillings are given on pages 76, 77, 94 and 95. Remember to add filling figures to pancake figures.

Each pancake contains 10g CHO and 60 calories.

Note: These pancakes freeze well empty, separated by layers of greaseproof paper. Fill after thawing.

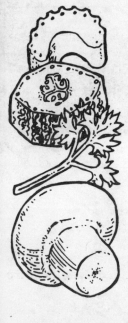

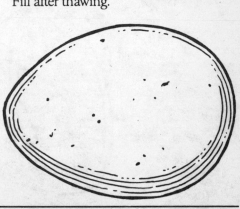

Kipper and Cheese Pancake Filling

Fills 8 pancakes   Total CHO — 20g   Total Cals — 675

8 oz (225g) kipper,
or smoked mackerel,
cooked and flaked
¼ pint (150ml) white
sauce (see page 26)
1 medium onion,
finely chopped
Sea salt and freshly
ground black pepper
1 tablespoon fresh
chopped parsley
1 tablespoon lemon
juice

Combine all the ingredients thoroughly.
Use with the pancake recipe on page 75.

Note: This recipe freezes well.

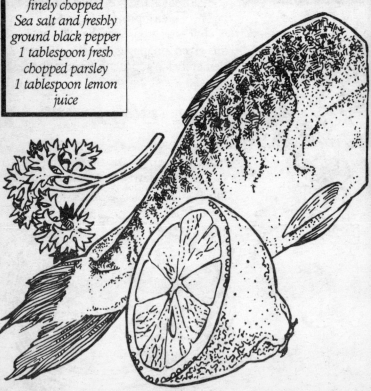

Savoury Vegetable Pancake Filling

Serves 1   Total CHO — neg   Total Cals — 25

1 oz (25g) mushrooms
1 oz (25g) pepper
(green or red)
1 oz (25g) courgette
1 oz (25g) celery
1 oz (25g) onion
¼ pint (150ml) water
1 tablespoon
tomato purée
½ teaspoon cornflour
Curry powder

1. Chop the vegetables finely.
2. Place in ¼ pint (150ml) boiling water and simmer for 5 minutes.
3. Add the purée, cornflour and curry powder and mix thoroughly. Use with the pancake recipe on page 75.

Note: This recipe freezes well.

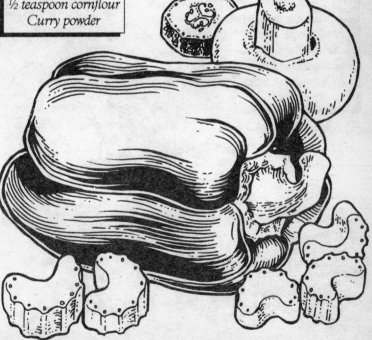

Cheesy Leeks and Ham

Serves 1   Total CHO — 35g   Total Cals — 440

*8 oz (225g) leeks,
washed and cut into
2-inch (5cm) lengths
1 oz (25g) low-fat
spread
1 tablespoon
wholemeal flour
¼ pint (150ml)
skimmed milk
Seasoning
1 oz (25g) reduced-fat
hard cheese, grated
1 oz (25g) wholemeal
breadcrumbs
2 slices lean cooked
ham*

1. Gently boil the leeks for 10 minutes. Drain well and keep warm.

2. Melt the low-fat spread, stir in the flour and cook for 2-3 minutes. Gradually add the milk and bring to the boil, stirring continuously. Simmer for 5 minutes, add cheese and seasoning.

3. Place the leeks in an ovenproof dish, cover with the ham and sauce and the breadcrumbs. Brown under the grill.

Note: This recipe is *not* suitable for freezing.

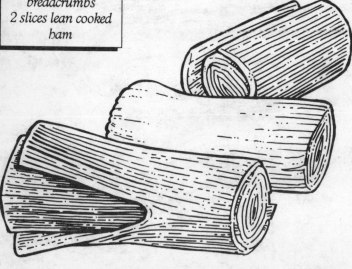

Pork Rissoles

Serves 1   Total CHO — 5g   Total Cals — 145

---

3 oz (75g) lean minced
pork
½ oz (15g) fresh
wholemeal
breadcrumbs
½ teaspoon French
mustard, ready-made
½ teaspoon tomato
purée
½ clove garlic, crushed
Sea salt and freshly
ground black pepper
Fresh parsley

1. Mix all the ingredients together well. Form into two rissoles.

2. Grill under a medium heat for 10 minutes on each side.

3. Garnish with parsley and sliced tomato. Serve with green salad.

Note: This recipe is *not* suitable for freezing.

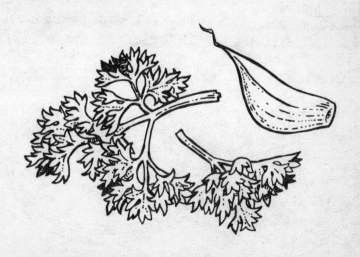

Mushroom Omelette

Serves 1	Total CHO — neg	Total Cals — 90

2 oz (50g) button mushrooms, sliced
3 fl oz (75ml) skimmed milk
Sea salt and freshly ground black pepper
2 × size 3 eggs, well beaten
1 teaspoon sunflower oil

1. Place the mushrooms in a saucepan with the milk, pepper and salt. Bring to the boil, reduce the heat and simmer with the lid on the pan for 10 minutes.

2. Whisk the eggs until fluffy. Heat the oil in an omelette pan and pour in the egg mixture. Cook slowly on a low heat for approximately 5 minutes.

3. When the eggs have set, add the drained mushrooms. Cook for a further 5 minutes on a medium heat. Fold the omelette over, remove from the pan and serve garnished with sliced red pepper rings and cress.

Note: This recipe is *not* suitable for freezing.

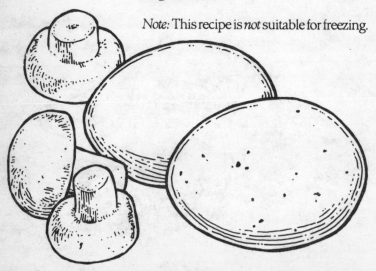

Sweet and Sour Eggs

Serves 1	Total CHO — 15g	Total Cals — 270

1 teaspoon oil
½ small onion, sliced
1 carrot, cut into thin strips
2 oz (50g) beansprouts
2 oz (50g) sweetcorn
1 oz (25g) mushrooms
2 tablespoons pineapple juice
1 teaspoon soya sauce
2 hard-boiled eggs (size 3)
Seasoning

1. Heat the oil. Gently sauté the onion and carrot and cook for 3 minutes. Add the vegetables and cook for 3 minutes, stirring continuously.

2. Add the pineapple juice and soya sauce. Season and heat through. Place vegetables on a plate and top with sliced eggs.

Note: This recipe is *not* suitable for freezing.

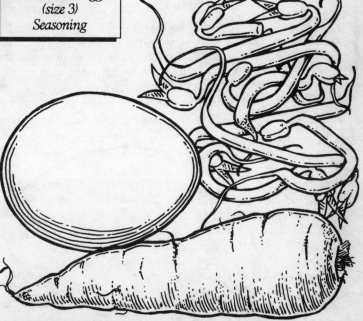

Curried Egg

Serves 1	Total CHO — 30g	Total Cals — 260

1½ oz (37g) long-grain brown rice
½ small onion
2 small mushrooms
1 rasher lean bacon
½ teaspoon wholemeal flour
A knob of low-fat spread
1 level teaspoon curry powder
A little stock
Seasoning
A hard-boiled egg (size 3)

1. Boil the rice in lightly salted water for 20 minutes.

2. Peel the onion and mushrooms and chop finely. Cut the bacon into strips, removing the rind first.

3. Heat the fat and sauté the onion until golden. Add the bacon and mushrooms to the pan and cook for a further few minutes. Mix the flour and curry powder with a little of the stock and add to the pan. Pour on the remaining stock and stir until the sauce thickens. Simmer for about 2 minutes and check for seasoning.

4. Cut the egg in half, arrange on a warmed serving dish and pour on the contents of the frying pan. Drain the rice and make a border round the egg mixture.

Note: This recipe is *not* suitable for freezing.

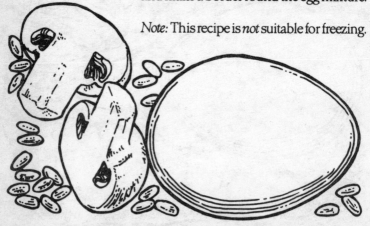

Spiced Liver

Serves 1	Total CHO — 5g	Total Cals — 160

3 oz (75g) lamb's liver,
thinly sliced
1 medium tomato,
deseeded and chopped
½ medium onion,
finely chopped
½ medium green
pepper, deseeded and
chopped
1 medium courgette,
sliced
3 fl oz (75ml) beef
stock
Sea salt and freshly
ground black pepper
1 clove of garlic,
crushed

1. Place all the ingredients in a large saucepan.
2. Bring to the boil, reduce the heat and simmer with the lid on the pan for 30 minutes. Garnish with fresh parsley.

Note: This recipe freezes well.

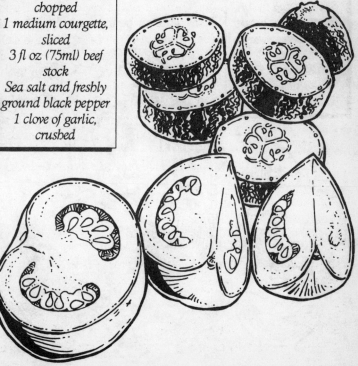

Liver Provençale

Serves 1	Total CHO — neg	Total Cals — 150

½ medium green pepper, deseeded and chopped
2 oz (50g) mushrooms, sliced
1 clove garlic, crushed
3 fl oz (75ml) vegetable stock
Sea salt and freshly ground black pepper
1 teaspoon mixed herbs
3 oz (75g) calves' liver, sliced
Juice of half a lemon

1. Place all the ingredients except the liver and lemon juice in a large saucepan. Bring to the boil, reduce the heat and simmer with the lid on the pan for 20 minutes.

2. Cover the liver with the lemon juice and grill for 8 minutes on each side. When cooked, place on a serving dish and pour over the vegetables. Serve immediately.

Note: This recipe freezes well.

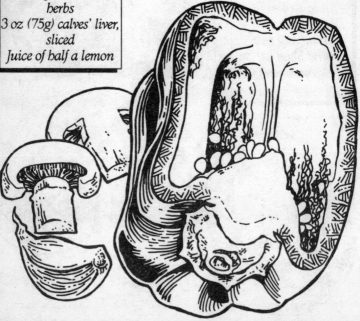

Liver Stroganoff

Serves 1	Total CHO — 20g	Total Cals — 300

4 oz (100g) pig's or lamb's liver, sliced
1 medium onion, finely chopped
1 tablespoon wholemeal flour
Sea salt and freshly ground black pepper
1 teaspoon vegetable oil
3 fl oz (75ml) skimmed milk
½ small carton natural yogurt
1 tablespoon lemon juice
1 tablespoon chopped parsley

1. Toss the liver in seasoned flour. Heat the oil and gently fry the liver and onion until golden brown. Gradually add the milk.
2. Cook slowly, stirring all the time, until the mixture thickens, then simmer for 5 minutes.
3. Stir in the yogurt and lemon juice. Spoon into a serving dish and garnish with chopped parsley.

Note: This recipe freezes well.

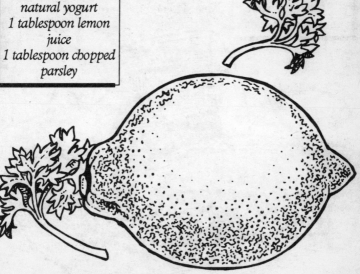

Spicy Vegetables

Serves 1	Total CHO — 10g	Total Cals — 180

1 tablespoon olive oil
½ small onion, finely
    chopped
½ green pepper, diced
1 small courgette,
    sliced
½ small aubergine,
    sliced *
1×5 oz (150g) can
    tomatoes and juice
1 bay leaf
1 clove garlic, crushed
A pinch of sea salt
½ teaspoon black
    pepper

1. Sprinkle the aubergine with salt. Leave it to stand for 1 hour, then wash it and pat dry.

2. Gently fry the onion in the oil, add the peppers and courgette, and fry for 2-3 minutes.

3. Add the remaining ingredients including the seasoning and simmer for 25 minutes.

* Use the other half in the Ratatouille on page 39.

Note: This recipe freezes well.

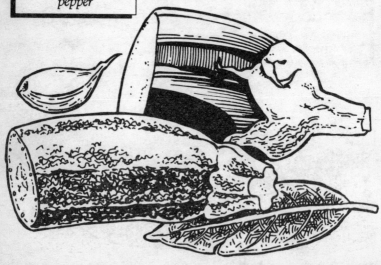

Courgettes and Red Pepper

Serves 1	Total CHO — 15g	Total Cals — 180

1 oz (25g) low-fat spread
8 oz (225g) courgettes, sliced
½ medium red pepper, deseeded and sliced
1 tablespoon tomato juice
2 teaspoons fresh parsley, chopped
2 teaspoons sultanas
¼ teaspoon celery salt
Freshly ground black pepper

1. Melt the spread in a large saucepan. Add the sliced courgettes, red pepper and tomato juice. Stir over a low heat for 3 minutes.
2. Add the parsley, sultanas, celery salt and black pepper to taste. Cover the pan, bring to the boil and cook for a further 3 minutes. Serve immediately.

Note: This recipe freezes well.

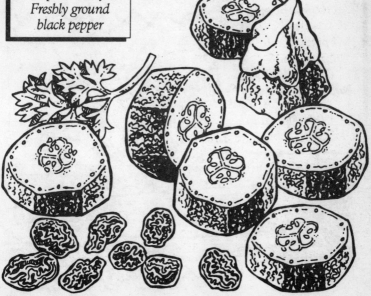

Kipper Lasagne

Makes 1 large or 2 small portions Total CHO — 55g Total Cals — 650

½ oz (15g) low-fat
spread
½ onion, chopped
1 stick celery, sliced
4 oz (100g) kipper,
skinned and flaked
1×5 oz (150g) can of
tomatoes, drained

Sauce
½ oz (15g) low-fat
spread
½ oz (15g) wholemeal
flour
¼ pint (150ml)
skimmed milk
1 oz (25g) reduced-fat
hard cheese, grated

2 oz (50g) wholegrain
lasagne, cooked

1. Melt the low-fat spread, sauté the onion and celery. Add the fish and tomatoes.
2. Place all the sauce ingredients in a pan. Bring to the boil, stirring well. Cook for 2 minutes.
3. Place alternate layers of lasagne, fish mixture and sauce in an ovenproof dish, ending with a layer of sauce. Brown under the grill for 5-10 minutes.

Note: This recipe freezes well.

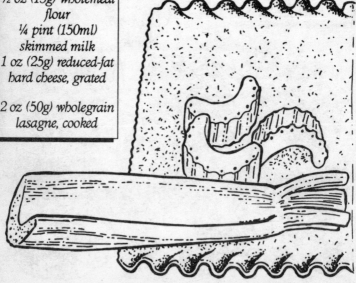

Brown Rice with Peppers, Mushroom and Onion

Serves 1	Total CHO — 40g	Total Cals — 210

2 oz (50g) brown rice
3 fl oz (75ml) water
2 oz (50g) onion, chopped
1 oz (25g) green pepper, chopped
1 oz (25g) red pepper, chopped
2 oz (50g) mushrooms
1 tablespoon tomato purée
Soya sauce

1. Boil the rice until tender.
2. Bring the 3 fl oz (75ml) of water to the boil.
3. Put the onion in the water and simmer until tender.
4. Add the peppers, mushrooms and tomato purée and simmer until tender.
5. Add soya sauce to taste.

Note: This recipe is not suitable for freezing.

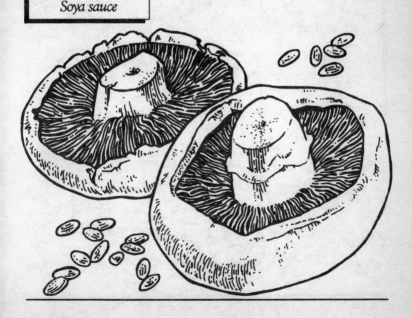

Brown Rice with Vegetables

Serves 1   Total CHO — 45g   Total Cals — 225

2 oz (50g) brown rice
3 fl oz (75ml) water
1 oz (25g) onion,
    chopped
1 oz (25g) beansprouts
1 oz (25g) peas
1 oz (25g) sweetcorn
1 tablespoon tomato
    purée
Seasoning

1. Boil the rice until tender.
2. Bring the 3 fl oz (75ml) of water to the boil.
3. Add the onion and cook until tender.
4. Add all the other vegetables and cook until tender.
5. Season to taste.

Note: This recipe is not suitable for freezing.

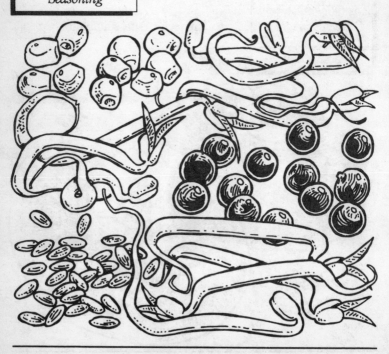

Cauliflower Cheese

Serves 1   Total CHO — 10g   Total Cals — 145

4 oz (100g) cauliflower in small pieces
2 teaspoons low-fat spread
2 teaspoons wholemeal flour
3 fl oz (75ml) skimmed milk
½ oz (15g) reduced-fat hard cheese, grated
Sea salt and freshly ground black pepper

1. Prepare the cauliflower and place in simmering water (with pan lid on) for 5 minutes or until tender.
2. Melt the low-fat spread.
3. Stir in the flour and cook for 1 minute.
4. Take off heat and stir in milk gradually, making sure there are no lumps.
5. Bring to the boil, stirring all the time.
6. Add the cheese and salt and pepper to the thickened sauce.
7. Simmer gently for 1 minute.
8. Drain the cooked cauliflower and pour the sauce over the top.
9. Serve hot.

Note: This recipe is *not* suitable for freezing.

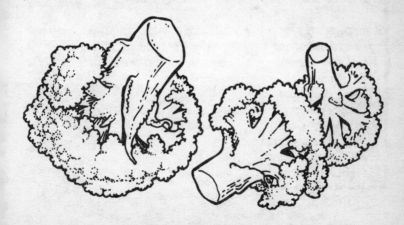

Broad Beans and Carrot

Serves 1   Total CHO — 5g   Total Cals — 35

3 fl oz (75ml) water
2 oz (50g) canned
broad beans
2 oz (50g) sliced carrot
Parsley

1. Bring 3 fl oz (75ml) of water to the boil.
2. Put in the vegetables and simmer for 10 minutes or until tender (with pan lid on).
3. Drain and serve, decorated with parsley.

Note: This recipe is *not* suitable for freezing.

Courgettes and Red Peppers

Serves 1   Total CHO — 15g   Total Cals — 180

1 oz (25g) low-fat
spread
½ lb (225g) courgettes,
sliced
½ medium red pepper,
deseeded and sliced
1 tablespoon tomato
juice
2 teaspoons fresh
parsley, chopped
2 teaspoons sultanas
¼ teaspoon celery salt
Freshly ground black
pepper to taste

1. Melt the spread in a large saucepan. Add the sliced courgettes, red pepper and tomato juice. Stir over a low heat for 3 minutes.
2. Add the parsley, sultanas, celery salt and pepper. Cover the pan, bring to the boil and cook for a further 3 minutes. Serve immediately.

Note: This recipe freezes well.

Broccoli and Almonds

Serves 1	Total CHO — neg	Total Cals — 150

3 fl oz (75ml) water
2 oz (50g) broccoli
1 teaspoon
polyunsaturated
margarine
1 oz (25g) almonds
(blanched)

1. Bring 3 fl oz (75ml) of water to the boil.
2. Put in the broccoli and simmer for 5 minutes or until tender (with the pan lid on).
3. Melt the margarine and sauté the almonds until golden brown.
4. Drain the broccoli and decorate with the almonds.

Note: This recipe is *not* suitable for freezing.

Courgettes and Celery

Serves 1	Total CHO — neg	Total Cals — 15

3 fl oz (75ml) water
2 oz (50g) sliced
courgette
2 oz (50g) sliced celery
Parsley

1. Bring 3 fl oz (75ml) water to the boil.
2. Add the vegetables and simmer for 5 minutes or until tender (with pan lid on).
3. Drain and decorate with parsley.

Note: This recipe is *not* suitable for freezing.

Fruit Salad and Lemon Pancake Filling

Fills 8 Pancakes with enough left for 1 plate of fruit salad
Total CHO — 250g   Total Cals — 950

*5 oz (150g) dried
prunes
5 oz (150g) dried
apricots
5 oz (150g) sultanas
6 fl oz (200ml) orange
juice
Rind of a lemon,
grated*

1. Soak dried fruit overnight in orange juice.

2. Stone the prunes and add the lemon rind. Simmer gently for approximately 10 minutes until liquid is thick and syrupy. Leave to cool.

Use with the pancake recipe on page 75.

Note: This recipe freezes well.

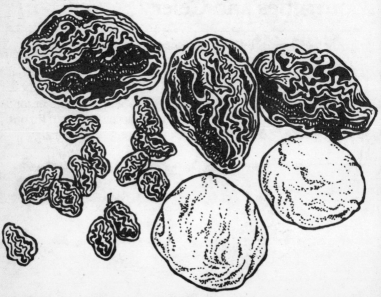

Spicy Apple Pancake Filling

Fills 8 pancakes   Total CHO — 40g   Total Cals — 180

1 lb (450g) cooking
apples, peeled and
diced
4 fl oz (100ml) orange
juice
1 teaspoon lemon juice
1 teaspoon mixed
spice
Liquid sweetener to
taste

1. Cook apples in fruit juice and spice for 15-20 minutes until the apple is of a thick sauce consistency.

2. Leave to cool and add sweetener to taste.

Use with the pancake recipe on page 75.

Note: This recipe freezes well.

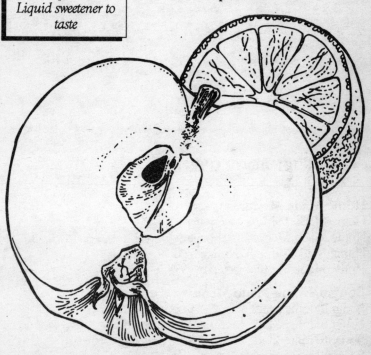

Custard

Serves 1   Total CHO — 15g   Total Cals — 90

---

*⅓ pint (180ml)
skimmed milk
2 teaspoons custard
powder
Liquid sweetener to
taste*

1. Make a paste from 2 tablespoons of the milk and custard powder.
2. Bring the rest of the milk to the boil. Pour into the paste.
3. Return to the pan and stir well. Bring to the boil, stirring continuously. Serve.

Note: This recipe is *not* suitable for freezing.

COLOUR PHOTOGRAPHS
(Next eight pages)

Home-Made Menus
Home-Made Menu 1 (see page 97)
Home-Made Menu 2 (see page 97)
Home-Made Menu 3 (see page 98)
Home-Made Menu 4 (see page 99)

Bought/Home-Made Menus
Bought/Home-Made Menu 1 (see page 98)
Bought/Home-Made Menu 2 (see page 98)
Bought/Home-Made Menu 3 (see page 99)
Bought/Home-Made Menu 4 (see page 99)

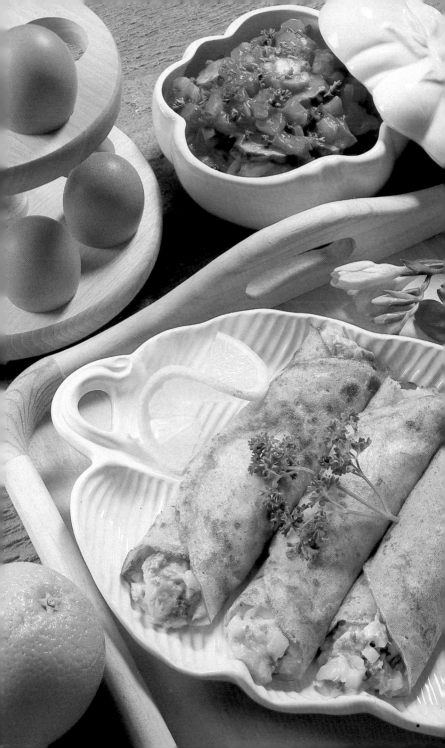

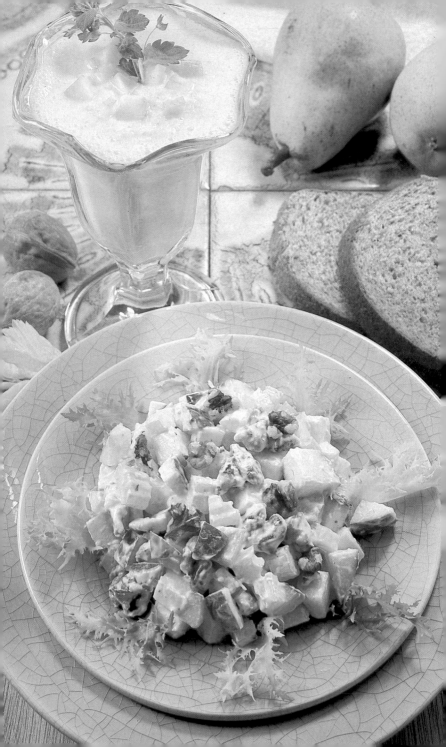

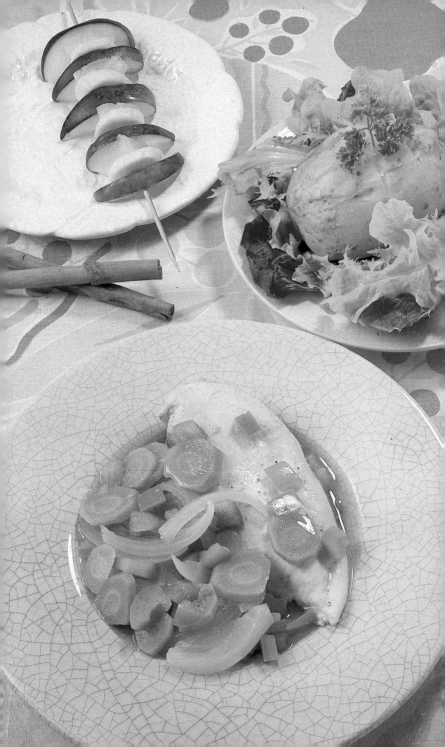

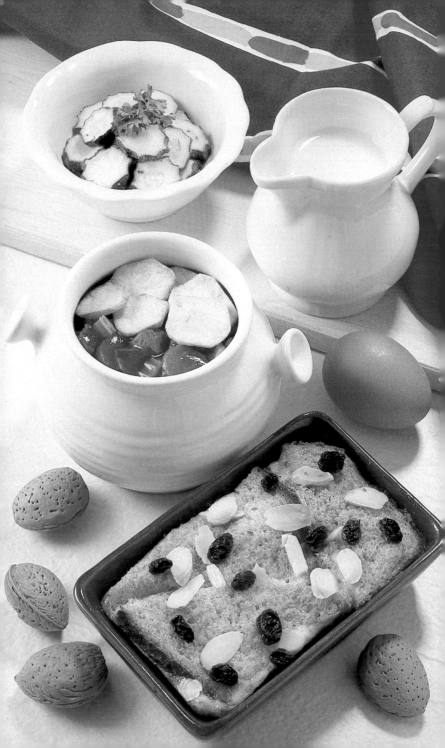

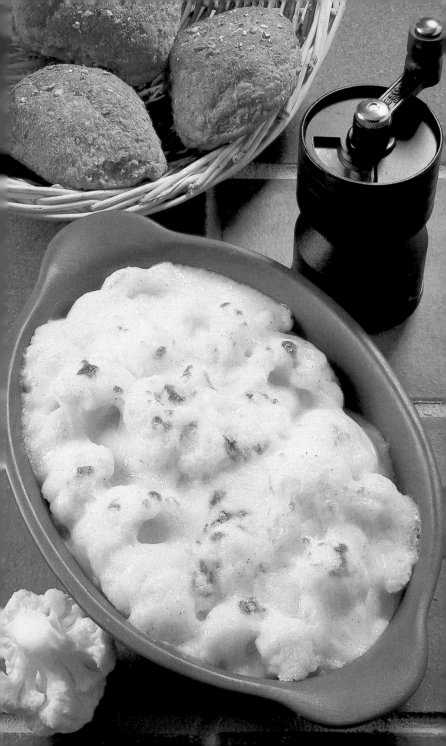

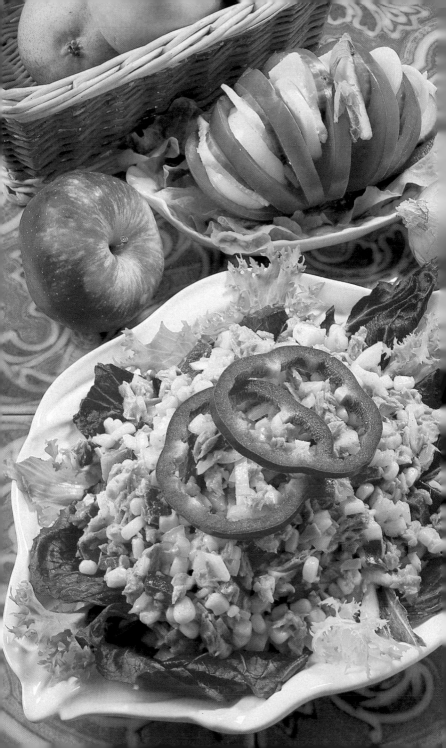

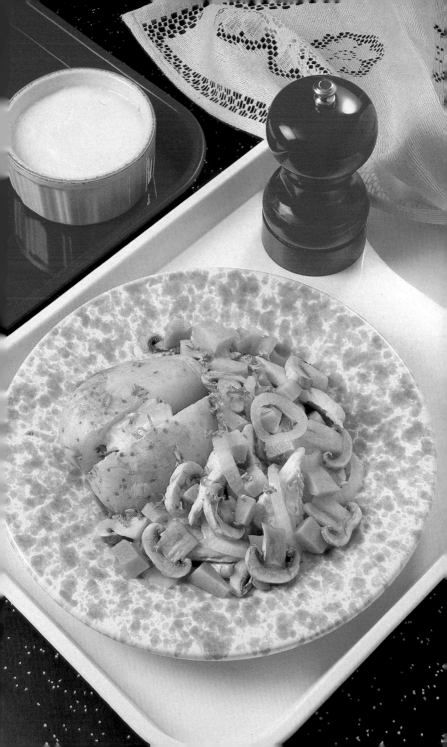

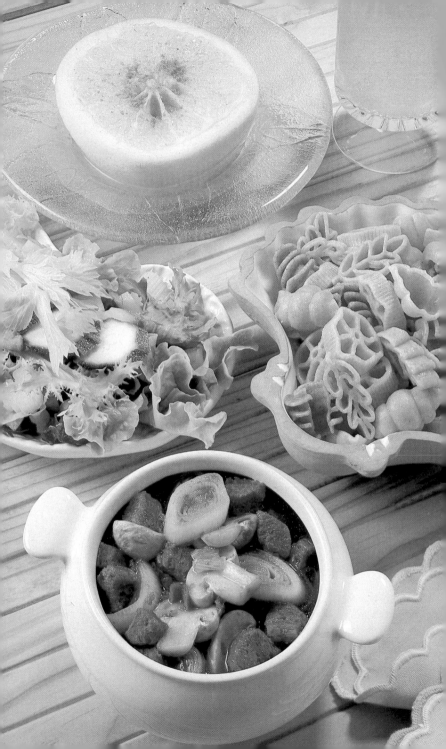

7. Menu Suggestions

It is important to remember that everyone has an individual diet plan which is aimed at providing an individual amount of carbohydrate and/or calories from which they must design their own meals. But it is sometimes helpful to have suggestions for possible menus. To give you some idea of the range of foods that can be enjoyed, I have produced a range of carbohydrate and calorie counted menus — which, of course, you can easily adapt to fit into your own particular circumstances.

Home-Made Menus

Four home-made meals for you to try.

MENU 1
A light lunch with 20g CHO and under 200 calories

	CHO	Cals
1 Pancake Parcel (page 75)	10g	60
1 portion Kipper and Cheese Filling (page 76)	—	85
1 orange	10g	40
	20g	185

MENU 2
A non-cook lunch with 30g CHO and 360 calories

	CHO	Cals
1 portion Waldorf Cheese Salad (page 61)	10g	240
1 slice wholemeal bread	15g	75
1 portion Fruit Wonder (page 71)	5g	45
	30g	360

MENU 3

A microwave meal with 40g CHO and just 300 calories

	CHO	Cals
1 portion Chicken and Vegetables (page 22)	5g	150
1×5 oz (150g) Jacket Potato (page 27)	25g	110
1 Hot Fruit Kebab (page 34)	10g	40
	40g	300

MENU 4

A meal using your oven, with 50g CHO and under 650 calories

	CHO	Cals
1 portion Hotpot (page 49)	25g	400
1 portion courgettes	—	25
1 portion Bread and Butter Pudding (page 59)	25g	220
	50g	645

Bought/Home-Made Menus

Healthy combinations of home-made and bought foods.

MENU 1

A light lunch with 20g CHO and under 200 calories

	CHO	Cals
1 portion Cauliflower Cheese (page 91)	10g	145
½ wholemeal roll	10g	50
	20g	195

MENU 2

A non-cook lunch with 30g CHO and under 500 calories

	CHO	Cals
1 Concertina Tomato (page 63)	5g	220
1 portion Tuna and Sweetcorn Salad (page 64)	15g	210
1 apple	10g	40
	30g	470

MENU 3

A meal using your oven, with 35g CHO and under 400 calories

	CHO	Cals
1 portion Chicken Casserole (page 52)	5g	150
1×5 oz (150g) Jacket Potato (cooked in the oven with Chicken Casserole for one hour) (page 27)	25g	110
1 Caramel Custard (page 56)	5g	125
	35g	385

MENU 4

A meal using your microwave, with 50g CHO and only 400 calories

	CHO	Cals
1 Ginger Grapefruit (page 35)	5g	25
1 portion Casseroled Pork (page 21)	10g	180
1 portion Pasta (page 24)	35g	160
Green salad	—	35
Diet fizzy drink	—	—
	50g	400

Appendix:
Food Values List

The carbohydrate and calorie contents of all the ingredients mentioned in the book are given so you can swap foods around and do a little experimenting of your own.

Food	Amount	gCHO	Cals
Almonds, ground	1 oz (25g)	1	160
Apple — eating, whole	1	10	40
cooking, raw	1 lb (450g)	35	140
Apricots, dried	1 oz (25g)	12	50
Aubergines, raw	1 lb (450g)	11	50
Bacon, lean shoulder	1 lb (450g)	—	670
Banana, raw	1 medium	10	40
Beans — Borlotti, tinned	1×15 oz (425g) tin	40	250
Butter, tinned	1×15 oz (425g) tin	50	280
Green, frozen	1 lb (450g)	18	120
Haricot, dry	1 oz (25g)	13	80
Kidney, tinned	1×15 oz (425g) tin	64	333
Beansprouts, raw	1 lb (450g)	10	50
Beef, steak, stewing, raw	1 lb (450g)	—	800
Blackberries, frozen, fresh	1 lb (450g)	30	130
Bread, wholemeal	1 oz (25g)	12	60
Broccoli	1 lb (450g)	10	105
Carrot, raw	1 lb (450g)	20	100
Cauliflower, raw	1 lb (450g)	7	60
Celery, raw	1 lb (450g)	5	30

Food	Amount	gCHO	Cals
Cheese — cottage	1 oz (25g)	neg	27
curd	1 oz (25g)	neg	40
reduced-fat, hard	1 oz (25g)	neg	80
reduced-fat, soft	1 oz (25g)	neg	40
Cider, dry	½ pint (275ml)	4	110
Coconut, desiccated	1 oz (25g)	1-2	170
Cod, fillet, raw	1 lb (450g)	—	345
Cornflour	1 oz (25g)	26	100
Courgettes, raw	1 lb (450g)	15	100
Cucumber, raw	1 lb (450g)	8	45
Currants, dried	1 oz (25g)	18	70
Custard, powder	1 oz (25g)	26	100
Eggs, raw	1×size 3	—	74
Flour — Wholemeal, plain	1 oz (25g)	18	90
Plain, white	1 oz (25g)	22	100
81% SR	1 oz (25g)	19	92
Fructose (fruit sugar)	1 oz (25g)	30*	115
Gelatine	1 sachet	—	35
Grapefruit, raw	1 lb (450g)	10	50
Ham, lean, boiled	1 oz (25g)	—	35
Kipper, fillet, raw	1 oz (25g)	—	60
Jam, low sugar	1 oz (25g)	8—10	30
Lamb — chop, lean	1 lb (450g)	—	1000
lean	1 lb 450g)	—	890
kidney	1 lb (450g)	—	410
Leeks, raw	1 lb (450g)	30	140
Liver, lambs, raw	1 lb (450g)	—	815
Low-fat spread	1 oz (25g)	—	105
Marmalade, low sugar	1 oz (25g)	8—10	30
Margarine, polyunsaturated	1 oz (25g)	—	210

* Note: Usually ignored if less than 1 oz (25g) taken in one day.

Food	Amount	gCHO	Cals
Mayonnaise, reduced-oil	1 tablespoon	neg	35
Milk — semi-skimmed	1 pint (550ml)	30	260
skimmed, dried	1 oz (25g)	15	100
skimmed, fresh	1 pint (550ml)	30	190
Muesli, unsweetened	1 oz (25g)	18	100
Mushrooms — raw	1 lb (450g)	—	70
soup	1×10 oz (275g) tin	11	150
Oats, raw	1 oz (25g)	20	110
Oil — olive	1 fl oz (25ml)	—	255
vegetable	1 fl oz (25ml)	—	255
Onion, raw	1 lb (450g)	25	100
Orange, raw	1	10	40
Orange juice, fresh, unsweetened	¼ pint (150ml)	15	60
Parsnip, raw	1 lb (450g)	40	160
Pasta, dry, wholegrain	1 oz (25g)	19	95
Pear, eating, raw	1	10	40
Peas, green	1 oz (25g)	3	20
Pepper, green/red, raw	1 lb (450g)	8	60
Pineapple, tinned in natural juice	1×15 oz (425g) tin	55	240
Pork, lean	1 lb (450g)	—	670
Potato, raw	1 lb (450g)	80	340
Raisins, dried	1 oz (25g)	18	70
Rice — brown, long grain	1 oz (25g)	21	105
white, ground	1 oz (25g)	24	102
Rum	1 fl oz (25ml)	neg	65
Sausage, pork	1	6	200
Sultanas, dried	1 oz (25g)	18	70
Sweetcorn, tinned	1×11 oz (300g) tin	55	250
Tomatoes — fresh	1 lb (450g)	10	60
juice, fresh, unsweetened	18 fl oz (1 litre)	40	190

Food	Amount	gCHO	Cals
Tomatoes, tinned	1×14 oz (405g) tin	10	50
Tuna in brine	1×7 oz (200g) tin	—	220
Turnip, raw	1 lb (450g)	15	90
Walnuts	1 oz (25g)	1½	150
Wholewheat flakes	1 oz (25g)	22	100
Wine, dry, white	4 fl oz (100ml)	2	85
Yogurt — natural, low-fat	1×5 oz (150g) pot	10	80
diet, fruit	1×4½ oz (125g) pot	7	55

Recommended Reading

These books contain lots of helpful information and recipes which you can use or adapt to suit one person.

Countdown
(Published by British Diabetic Association)
A guide to carbohydrate and calorie content of manufactured foods.

Better Cookery for Diabetics
(Published by British Diabetic Association)
A recipe book by Jill Metcalfe.

Cooking the New Diabetic Way
(Published by British Diabetic Association)
A recipe book by Jill Metcalfe.

Simple Diabetic Cookery
(Published by British Diabetic Association)
A recipe leaflet.

Simple Home Baking
(Published by British Diabetic Association)
A recipe leaflet by Sue Hall.

The Vegetarian on a Diet
(Published by Thorsons Publishing Group, 1984)
A recipe book for vegetarians by Margaret Cousins and Jill Metcalfe.

The Diabetic's Microwave Cookbook
(Published by Thorsons Publishing Group, 1986)
A microwave book by Sue Hall.

Cooking for Diabetes
(Published by Thorsons Publishing Group, 1985)
A recipe book by Jill Metcalfe.

Knowing about Diabetes (1) for Insulin Dependent Diabetics; (2) for Non-Insulin Dependent (Maturity Onset) Diabetics
(Published by W. Fowlsham and Co. 1983)
By P. H. Wise.

Diet and Diabetes (Patient Handbook 21)
(Published by Churchill Livingstone)
By Briony Thomas.

The Diabetes Handbook
Non-Insulin Dependent Diabetes
(Published by Thorsons Publishing Group, 1986)
By Dr John Day.

The Diabetes Handbook
Insulin Dependent Diabetes
(Published by Thorsons Publishing Group, 1986)
By Dr John Day.

Packed Lunches and Snacks
(Published by Thorsons Publishing Group, 1986)
A recipe book by Sue Hall.

One is Fun!
(Published by Guild Publishing, 1985)
A recipe book (not Diabetic) by Delia Smith.

Further Information

BRITISH DIABETIC ASSOCIATION
Diabetes affects just over two per cent of the UK population.
Although it cannot be cured or prevented, it can be controlled by
proper treatment.

The *British Diabetic Association* (BDA) was formed in 1934 to help
all diabetics, to overcome prejudice and ignorance about diabetes,
and to raise money for research. The Association is currently
budgeting over £1.5m each year to treat, prevent or cure diabetes,
and is the largest single contributor to diabetic research in the UK.

The Association is an independent organization with over 100,000
members and 350 local branches. It provides information and advice
for diabetics and their families. It also liaises closely with those
who work in the field of diabetes.

Educational and activity holidays are organized for diabetics of
all ages plus teach-in weekends for families with diabetic children
or teenagers.

The BDA's bi-monthly magazine *Balance* keeps readers up to
date with news of the latest research and all aspects of diabetes.
It is sent free to members or available from local newsagents, price
85p.

All diabetics have to follow a lifelong diet and *Balance* publishes
recipes and dietary information to help bring interest and variety
to eating.

To become a member, fill in the application form and send it with your subscription to:

British Diabetic Association,
10 Queen Anne Street,
London W1M 0BD.
Tel: 01-323 1531

Enrolment Form

The British Diabetic Association
10 Queen Anne Street
London W1M 0BD

MEMBERSHIP SUBSCRIPTIONS

Life membership	Single payment of £105 or £15 a year for 7 years under covenant
Annual membership	£5.00 a year
Reduced membership — pensioner, student on Government grant and those in receipt of DHSS benefits	£1.00 a year
Overseas annual membership	£10.00 a year
Overseas life membership	Single payment of £150.00

Please enrol me as a:

☐ Life member: £105 £15 a year for 7 years under covenant

☐ Annual member: £5.00

☐ Pensioner member: £1.00

☐ Overseas annual member: £10.00

☐ Overseas Life member: £150.00

☐ Are you joining on behalf of a child? (Children in the UK under the age of 16 can join free for one year if they wish)

I enclose Remittance/Banker's Order/Covenant for £ ....
(Please delete whichever does not apply)

Date.................................Signature..........................

Full name: Mr/Mrs/Miss.....................................
(Block Capitals please)

Address ....

....

Date of Birth.........................Occupation..................
(This information will be treated as strictly confidential)

Index

Apple and Blackberry Crumble, 58
Apple, Baked Stuffed, 34
Apple Charlotte, 58
Apple Pancake Filling, Spicy, 95

Bacon and Sweetcorn Soup, Slow, 36
Bakewell Tart, 60
Banana Crunch, 33
Bananas, Juicy, 57
Beanfeast Soup, 74
Beansprout and Chicken Salad, Fruity, 66
Bread and Butter Pudding, 59
Broad Beans and Carrot, 92
Broccoli and Almonds, 93
Brown Betty, 57

Caramel Custard, 56
Cauliflower Cheese, 91
Cheesecake, 73
Cheese Salad, Waldorf, 61
Chicken and Beansprouts, 22
Chicken and Vegetables, 22
Chicken Casserole, 52
Chicken Curry and Rice, Quick, 41
Chicken Fillet, Spiced, 53
Chicken, Lemony, 43

Chicken Salad, Garlic, 65
Chicken, Slow-Cook Oriental, 38
Chicken, Slow Curried, 37
Chicken, Yogurt, 54
Corn, Pepper and Beansprout Salad, 62
Courgettes and Celery, 93
Courgettes and Red Pepper, 87
Custard, 96

Egg, Curried, 82
Egg Custard, Baked, 31
Eggs, Sweet and Sour, 81

Fish 'n' Beans, 23
flour, 13
fructose (fruit sugar), 14
Fruit Compote, 32
Fruit Crunch, 70
Fruit, Dried, Salad, 47
Fruit Fluff, 72
Fruit Kebabs, Hot, 34
Fruit Salad and Lemon Pancake Filling, 94
Fruit Wonder, 71
Fruit Yogurt Ice Cream, 72

Grapefruit, Ginger, 35

Ham and Haricot Bean Salad, 68
hints for solo cooking, 17

Hot Pot, 49

Kipper and Cheese Pancake
    Filling, 76
Kipper Kedgeree, 55
Kipper Lasagne, 88

Lamb, Marmalade, 45
Leeks and Ham, Cheesy, 78
Liver and Borlotti Beans, 44
Liver and Onions, Slow, 40
Liver, Mexican, 24
Liver Provencale, 84
Liver, Spiced, 83
Liver Stroganoff, 85
low-fat spread, 13

Madeleines, Individual, 48
Mushroom Cod, 46

Omelette, Mushroom, 80
Orange, Surprise, 70

Pancake Parcels, 75
Pasta in Your Microwave, 24
Pasta, Last-Minute, 25
Pasta Supper, Spicy, 42
Pears, Slow-Cook Lime and
    Ginger, 39
Pork and Butter Bean Casserole,
    19
Pork, Casseroled, 21
Pork Chop, Spicy, 51
Pork, Mushroomed, 20
Pork Rissoles, 79
Porridge, Fruity, 35
Potato, Cheesy Jacket, 29

Potato, Ham and Mushroom
    Jacket, 30
Potato, Jacket, 27
Potato, Vegetable Jacket, 28
Potatoes, Boiled, 31

Ratatouille, 39
Rice, Brown, with Peppers,
    Mushroom and Onion, 89
Rice, Brown, with Vegetables, 90
Rice in Your Microwave, 26
Rice Pudding, Traditional, 59
Rum, Raisin and Apricot Yogurt,
    69

Sauce, Cheese, 27
    White, 26
Sausage Goulash, 50

Tomato, Concertina, 63
Tuna and Spring Carrot Salad, 67
Tuna and Sweetcorn Salad, 64

Upside-Down Pudding, 33

Vegetable Mix, Crunchy, with
    Cottage Cheese, 69
Vegetable Pancake Filling,
    Savoury, 77
Vegetable Salad, Chinese, 63
Vegetable, Spicy, 86

West Country Chop, 52

Yogurt, 40
Yogurt Jelly, 71